Praise for Samir Becic and
ReSYNC Your Life

"Samir's new book, *ReSYNC Your Life*, is for everyone. It is customized to the individual, from the highly-trained athlete to the person who has just decided to become more fit. What's great is no equipment or machines are required, you can perform these exercises in the privacy of your home or just about any place. Do the workouts alone or with a partner. The exercises are clearly explained and well-illustrated. He has developed a versatile system that everyone can benefit from. I highly recommend this book."

—RUDY TOMJANOVICH, FORMER COACH OF THE HOUSTON ROCKETS AND LOS ANGELES LAKERS

"To simply label Samir Becic a fitness expert is egregiously limiting. Samir is the new global champion of modern well-being. His larger than life intensity is mirrored by his passion to revolutionize the world into a new health and fitness paradigm—a transformative revolution he hopes will help save humankind from itself. And he's wanting to assist us in that mission with every fiber of his being."

—MATT BALLESTEROS, CHIEF EXECUTIVE OFFICER OF SIX FOOT ENTERTAINMENT

"We spend billions in medication, surgeries and treatments to tackle life threatening health problems like diabetes, high blood pressure and heart disease. Spend a few bucks on this book, put the information to work and, chances are, these health issues will never be a problem!"

—DEBORAH DUNCAN, EMMY AWARD-WINNING HOST OF *GREAT DAY HOUSTON*

"Your body, brain, and spirit are all connected. Fitness guru Samir Becic has found a way to enhance each of them through a focused, engaging, and strategic plan in *ReSYNC Your Life*. In Houston and across the country, Samir is a fitness role model. My hope for the readers of *ReSYNC Your Life* is that they are motivated to read, get active, and commit to a healthier lifestyle, one day at a time."

—SYLVESTER TURNER, MAYOR OF HOUSTON

"When it comes to health and fitness, one name stands out, Samir Becic. An expert in his field, his passion is clear, his intelligent approach to healthy lifestyle made him unique and should be an inspiration to us all. *Resync Your Life* is a treat for body, mind, and spirit."

—Princess Tatiana Galitzine

"If you're not living the life you were meant to live, then you need to 'Resync' it. Samir Becic puts together, in four easy silos, how to get your strength, health, mind, and spirit back. He is a combination of Jack LaLanne with easy-to-do—in any location—exercises and Arnold Schwarzenegger with the determination and drive that it takes to achieve your goals. Know this . . . your life will get better as you get better."

—Peter C. Remington, publisher of *Modern Luxury* magazine

"I have known and trained with Samir for over six years. I can enthusiastically testify to Samir's unparalleled skills as a trainer. Samir has changed my life, and the life of my family. He is knowledgeable, enthusiastic, and single-minded in his commitment to the health, fitness, well-being, and the success of every person he works with. His innovative methods, together his infectious and indomitable personality, produce spectacular results in the face of the most challenging situations. Those that are lucky enough to train with Samir know that he has earned, and continues to earn every day, the honor of being named the best fitness trainer in the world."

—Robert J. Madden, JD

"I have seen Samir Becic in action and I endorse his book! People need to get with the Health Fitness Revolution."

—Lou Savarese, former heavyweight world champion

resync®
Your Life

resync®
Your Life
28 DAYS
TO A STRONGER, LEANER,
SMARTER, HAPPIER YOU

SAMIR BECIC

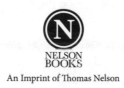

NELSON
BOOKS
An Imprint of Thomas Nelson

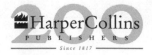

© 2017 by Samir Becic

Published in Nashville, Tennessee, by Nelson Books, an imprint of Thomas Nelson. Nelson Books and Thomas Nelson are registered trademarks of HarperCollins Christian Publishing, Inc.

ReSYNC® is a registered trademark of Samir Becic. Used with permission.

All photos were taken by Bryan Anderson. Used with permission.

Thomas Nelson titles may be purchased in bulk for educational, business, fund-raising, or sales promotional use. For information, please e-mail SpecialMarkets@ThomasNelson.com.

Unless otherwise noted, Scripture quotations are taken from the King James Version. Public domain.

Scripture quotations marked NIV are from the Holy Bible, New International Version®, NIV®. Copyright © 1973, 1978, 1984, 2011 by Biblica, Inc.® Used by permission of Zondervan. All rights reserved worldwide. www.Zondervan.com. The "NIV" and "New International Version" are trademarks registered in the United States Patent and Trademark Office by Biblica, Inc.˙

Any Internet addresses, phone numbers, or company or product information printed in this book are offered as a resource and are not intended in any way to be or to imply an endorsement by Thomas Nelson, nor does Thomas Nelson vouch for the existence, content, or services of these sites, phone numbers, companies, or products beyond the life of this book.

ISBN 978-0-7180-8990-0 (eBook)

Library of Congress Cataloging-in-Publication Data

ISBN 978-0-7180-8988-7
Names: Becic, Samir, 1976- author.
Title: ReSYNC your life : 28 days to a stronger, leaner, smarter, happier you / by Samir Becic.
Description: Nashville, Tennessee : Thomas Nelson, 2017. | Includes
   bibliographical references.
Identifiers: LCCN 2017006565 | ISBN 9780718089887 (hardback)
Subjects: LCSH: Physical fitness. | Physical fitness--Psychological aspects. | Nutrition. | Mental health. |
   Well-being.
Classification: LCC GV481 .B1955 2017 | DDC 613.7--dc23 LC record available at https://lccn.loc.
gov/2017006565

Printed in the United States of America

17 18 19 20 21   LSC   10 9 8 7 6 5 4 3 2 1

I dedicate this book to you, my readers.

Contents

My Promise to You

Some of us are not content to remain static.

Some of us are not content to grow older, heavier, weaker, and more
    confused.

Some of us refuse to give in to the ravages of time.

Some of us want to make more of what we have been given in this life.

We want to be strong. We want to be lean. We want to be smart. We want
    to be happy.

Some of us know that our bodies are made for this,

but to achieve it, we need to resynchronize.

Some of us know that our minds can achieve this,

but to make it happen, we need to reprogram.

Some of us know that our spirits long for this,

but to find it, we need a battle plan.

Some of us know that health is our destiny,

and we will fight for it,
if we have a method.

Hey, you. Yes, you. I have something very important to tell you.

I am on a mission, and my mission concerns *you*. My mission is a matter of life and death. How well I accomplish my mission could affect the political course of history, the financial success of our nation, the crime rates that plague our cities, and the personal health and happiness of every citizen of the world. If I fail, the consequences could be dire on a grand scale. My mission is nothing less than revolutionary, but my mission parameters are simple: Get you healthy. Get you fit. Get you smart. Get you happy again. But this will require some reprogramming. Why? Because your body is in rapid decline. You are prematurely aging—both your body and your mind—because of an unhealthy lifestyle, and as a result you are feeling unhappy, unhealthy, and unfulfilled. But it doesn't have to be this way.

I want to change the world, one person at a time, and I want to start with you.

Yes, you. I am here to help you get better. The human body was designed to be lean, strong, smart, and happy. We were created to have an abundance of natural energy to live our lives. Our ancestors required energy to survive, and if we had continued the diets and lifestyles they practiced, then with all our modern advances, we would be much healthier than we are now. Instead, civilization has gotten the best of us. But it's not too late. In fact, I will show you how you can functionally reverse the aging process. The longer you use the ReSYNC Method, the younger your body will be. You will look younger, feel younger, and move and think like a younger person—but in reality, you will look, feel, move, and think the way you *should for your age*. Once you have reset your body and mind, you will be able to age efficiently and optimally; you will feel as if you have turned back the clock.

And that's when the real changes start. That's when you become more productive, more creative, more active, and more capable of doing good things for yourself, your family, and the world. That's when you can really start improving who you are and finding what you were meant to do with this body and this life. This is how you were always intended to live. I believe the ReSYNC Method could make the world more peaceful and more productive and virtually extinguish the stress, frustration, depression, and anger that plague so many. It could launch us into a future that is entirely different from the one we are headed toward now. All we have to do—all *you* have to do—is begin.

I know that you have potential beyond your imagination, and I have a mission for you. Your mission, should you choose to accept it, is to resynchronize your body, your mind, and your spirit so that you can finally achieve your vast human potential. You will show your boss, your employees, your teachers, your students, your colleagues, and your friends exactly what human beings can achieve.

No matter what your current state of health or physical ability, you can become what you were created to become.

I don't want you—and will never ask you—to do anything you cannot do or anything that will injure you or put you at risk. No gimmicks. No promises I can't guarantee. Just proven results. Major transformation starts with small steps. I will only ask you to make some adjustments that work for your unique self so that you can gradually change your own body and mind to become a little bit fitter, healthier, and smarter every day, without pain or unreasonable sacrifice. You can do this. I know you can.

But to be a part of this revolution will take resolve. It will take commitment. It won't always be easy, but the rewards will be significant.

Are you in?

INTRODUCTION

My Revolutionary Road

*Physical fitness is not only one of the most
important keys to a healthy body, it is the basis of
dynamic and creative intellectual activity.*
—JOHN F. KENNEDY

I was born in Bosnia and grew up in Germany. My journey starts with me as a thirteen-year-old boy working out on the balcony of our house at night so I wouldn't disturb my parents. My heroes at the time were Albert Einstein and Julius Caesar, as well as Bruce Lee, Chuck Norris, and Muhammad Ali.

When I was twenty-four years old, I was given the opportunity to come to the United States and received a green card, which gave me permanent residency status. My sponsoring program assigned me to Houston, Texas, where I began working out at a local Bally Total Fitness facility. One day I was spotted by a supervisor, who offered me a job as a trainer, and I readily accepted. At the time, I considered it a temporary stop on my career path, but within a year I was promoted to director and then to senior director, in charge of five clubs. After training several hundred other Bally fitness trainers and receiving several awards, including Bally's best fitness trainer, I left the company in 2009 to go out on my own.

When I first came to the United States in 2000, I, like many people who come to live in this country, had a preconceived view of America. I thought of it as the strongest financial and military power in the world, with a democracy and freedom unmatched by any other nation. I also imagined that every citizen would be the epitome of that success—strong and healthy, intelligent and motivated. But what I observed after living here was that, yes, we are strong in many ways, but we are also a nation of many unhealthy, inactive, junk food–addicted people. How did this happen to the greatest nation in the world?

The more I recognized this trend toward inactivity and poor nutrition, the more disturbed I became. I felt as though I was watching a superstar athlete waste his or her talent by refusing to practice, or a genius philosopher who insisted on sitting on a couch, watching TV all day, instead of reading and writing and formulating ideas. I could see the problem, and as a health and fitness expert, I thought I could see the solution. I decided that I had to do something about it. So I decided to devise my own American dream: I want this nation to lead the world in healthy lifestyles and physical fitness. Other countries already look to us as an example, so imagine the impact we can make if we commit to becoming healthy—in body, mind, and spirit. It is my hope that we can show the world a brighter, more positive future—one in which humans become better than they are today.

All living things change and adjust to their environments. If we are going to change for the better, we need to shape our environments toward that goal—and not fall into a downward spiral of obesity, depression, and chronic disease. Who do we want to be? What do we want to become? It's time to make a decision and move in the right direction, before it's too late.

Today more than a third of Americans are obese, and almost 75 percent are overweight. That translates to more than 250 million Americans! In my own state of Texas, the obesity rate is currently 61 percent, and just a few years ago, Houston, where I live, was named the fattest city in the nation. These are not points of pride for our great country, and the problem isn't one of mere vanity. Americans are experiencing chronic diseases like never before, costing the US economy more than $1 trillion every year. About 360,000 people die every year as a direct result of obesity, and millions more die every year due to causes that are indirectly connected to obesity and an unhealthy lifestyle. Texas spends roughly $5.7 billion on obesity-related chronic conditions such as hypertension, some cancers, type 2 diabetes, back problems, high cholesterol, and mental health issues, including depression and anxiety. The future looks bleak as well—34 percent of American children (40 percent of children in Texas) are overweight or obese, and many children are now being diagnosed with type 2 diabetes, not to mention depression, attention deficit hyperactivity disorder (ADHD), and other mental health problems. All of us, children and adults alike, eat a diet made up largely of fat and sugar with minimal nutrients and have become sedentary to the point of madness.

We must turn this around. The cost of looking the other way and doing nothing could far exceed the price we've paid in the past for world wars, natural disasters, and political conflicts. And yet this is a price we don't have to pay. This is a war we can win. This is an enemy we can defeat. But to make a change, we have little choice but to start a revolution.

Because I believe so strongly in our ability to do that, in 2011 I created a magazine called Health Fitness Revolution (www.healthfitnessrevolution.com) that gathers and publishes information about health and fitness, even tying in areas of politics, religion, and education—the first source to do so.

What if our country collectively decided to prioritize and champion physical fitness, healthy nutrition, and mental balance? I believe we could control, manage, or completely avoid 60 to 70 percent of known chronic diseases, including obesity. We would be a sharper, quicker, stronger nation with minds that excel and bodies that remain energetic and mobile far into old age. These healthy changes would contribute positively to every aspect of our great country—our financial health, our military strength, our very freedom. Why are we making excuses? What are we waiting for? The world is looking to us.

Bodies are meant to move, not to stay static. Muscles are meant to be used, and movement keeps both the body and the brain younger, more agile, more focused, and happier. I want to bring my message to every household in the country, and to the rest of the world too: you can feel better almost immediately. You don't have to get sick or live with fatigue and pain. You can have a fitter family and children who never have to struggle with weight issues or many of the chronic health conditions that come from a sedentary lifestyle and poor nutrition. You can be strong and smart, with a clear mind and boundless energy. You will work better and be more successful and financially secure if you are healthy and fit. You will set a strong example for your children if you are healthy and fit. You will feel better about yourself, have more confidence, and enjoy more energy if you are healthy and fit. You will be safer, faster, smarter, and savvier about who you are and how you should live when you are healthy and fit. By joining the Health Fitness Revolution and committing to the ReSYNC Method, you can achieve not just health but the fruition of all your potential.

Life is better with health. It is more complete, vivid, and full. How can anyone become a personal success, achieve as an athlete, be a great CEO, lead a congregation, or be a role model without health? How can anyone be the best possible boss or employee, teacher or student, parent or caregiver, partner or best friend without health? How can anyone be who they are truly meant to be without a body and a brain working at full potential?

I am not cynical about our future. I am an optimist, and I believe that with the right motivation and guidance, every single one of us can become better, and that starts with health. Health is the basis for a successful life. The old saying that if you don't have your health, you don't have anything is exactly right. And the way to achieve health is through fitness, good nutrition, and mental balance. If we want it, we can have it. We just need to stand up and take it. We just have to be extreme about balance.

I love this country, and not just because I was born on July 4, 1976, exactly two hundred years after the United States declared its independence. I love it because I see the potential this country has to powerfully lead the rest of world with inspiration and motivation. But being from Europe and having also lived and taught in Latin America, I know that leadership potential can be found in other countries. We are a planet of humans who have more in common than we have differences, and every one of us has the ability to improve. But to do this, many of us will need to change our ways. I'm not asking you to get up right now and run five miles. I'm asking you to start where you are and take small steps, one at a time, toward a better future for yourself, your family, your community, your country, and your world.

This is a global effort. A global revolution. And if we succeed, it could change the entire course of history. If we each embrace this mission and step into the future together, becoming shining examples of the next wave of humanity, we can solve any problem, and the future can be anything we want it to be.

Learn the ReSYNC Method

Every revolution needs a strategy, and the ReSYNC Method is the strategy I have developed to make health and fitness accessible to everyone. Every aspect of the program is adaptable to any person, requires no equipment, and can be accomplished at home. The nutrition plan uses foods available at any grocery store or supermarket, and the benefits will be dramatic and swift. I may be known for my extreme push-ups and running with a weighted vest of two hundred pounds or more, but the ReSYNC Method I developed as a full transformational program for the body and mind is not about being able to do push-ups or pull-ups or having six-pack abs or big biceps or perfect thighs (although these things are achievable too, if you really want them).

Instead, my method synchronizes every part of you—physical, intellectual, and spiritual. For more than fifteen years, I have been developing and refining key methods and techniques to meld these three components into one with the goal of synergizing your system in ways you've never experienced before. You will be better than you are right now. You will still be you, but a better you, a stronger, sharper, smarter, quicker, new-and-improved you.

The power of the ReSYNC Method comes from its simplicity—all you need to achieve personal acceleration is your own body. Every muscle in the body can be trained by the body's own movement and natural resistance, which makes this method a perfect option for all ages, sizes, and abilities. It can be adapted to accommodate any issue, from a sprained ankle to a missing limb, and it can be easily understood and practiced by anyone. You can change your body by simply using it—no gimmicks, equipment, or false promises. However, if you like exercise equipment, the method can be adapted for the gym, and I will also show you some signature ReSYNC exercises to do with partners or workout companions. Try them if you have someone working out with you. The ReSYNC Method shows you how to manipulate your own body weight to build strength and endurance in the physique, the brain, and the soul. Your mind and body will remake themselves.

The ReSYNC Method begins with a test to determine your current level of health, then prescribes a set of simple exercises that employ the brain and the body and a nutrition plan that is easy and satisfying to follow. As you become more physically fit, you will find that you are also becoming more spiritually balanced. There is a positive synergy between the physical and the spiritual.

It takes just four weeks to change your path, but it takes a lifetime to become who you were meant to be. The first twenty-eight days will "ReSYNC" you, and after that I will tell you how to stay "SYNCed" for the rest of your life.

CHAPTER 1

The Mission: To ReSYNC Your Body, Brain, and Spirit for a Longer, Healthier Life

Certainly there have been many programs created by trainers who want to make you fit, diets developed by nutritionists to help you eat healthier, studies by scientists on how to boost your brainpower, and guidance from spiritual leaders on how to be more fulfilled and content. What makes the ReSYNC Method different from all of these is that each of its four components—physical fitness, nutritional health, mental sharpness, and spiritual balance—work in synergy so that every aspect of your life begins to improve immediately and ensures that you will not only live longer but also better. You will experience more harmony and peace within yourself and with the world around you.

What Makes the ReSYNC Exercise Program Unique

You can do the ReSYNC exercise program anywhere—in a small space, even in a hotel room when you're traveling—and you don't need any equipment because the exercises I've developed use gravity and your own body weight to create resistance. When you squat, for example, gravity is pulling you down, and with each repetition, holding the squat and returning to a standing position becomes increasingly difficult.

The entry-level workout, which is where most people begin, takes just ten minutes. I know that doesn't sound like much, but that's the beauty of the program. Because you never stop, it's dynamic, combining strength training with mobility with flexibility, and it gets all your muscles working together at one time. That's why you are able to accomplish so much in so little time. And you also save the time it would take you to get to the gym, change your clothes, shower at the end of your workout, change clothes again, and get to the day's next activity.

Who do you think are the fittest athletes in the world? I'll tell you: elite tennis players. When you play tennis on the elite level, you're working every part of your body at the same time. If you've ever seen a five-set match between two of the world's best players, you probably got tired just watching. They move forward and backward, from side to side, running, jumping, squatting, and swinging their arms for three hours or more with little rest. Players change sides after every two games and have just ninety seconds from the end of one point to get to the other end of the court and begin the next point. At the end of each set, they get two minutes before starting the next set.

While the ReSYNC exercise program may not lead to your becoming an elite tennis player, it will work your muscles in much the same way that the sport at a high-performance level does. Most exercises work one muscle or one muscle group at a time, but that's not how muscles work in daily life. To do everyday things, such as moving the sofa to vacuum behind it, our muscles need to move in synchrony with one another. If they don't, we're more likely to injure ourselves. The ReSYNC Method prepares you to accomplish such practical activities as efficiently and painlessly as possible.

But what about going to the gym and working out on all those machines? Wouldn't that get you fitter faster? The answer is no. As a former fitness director for Bally Total Fitness, I was in charge of buying the machines for the facilities. I taught more than a thousand trainers how to use them, and I can tell you that machines are not the most effective way to go. When you're working out on a machine, you are using only a limited range of motion; your body actually becomes very static. When you use the ReSYNC Method, however, your body becomes more flexible, and you are moving more naturally, which means that you are also about 200 percent less likely to injure yourself than you are when using a machine.

A variation of the ReSYNC exercise program is partner training. I'll show you how to adapt the exercises so that they're easily done with a training partner, such as a sibling, spouse, or friend. When you train with a partner, you form a connection with that person, not only through the shared experience, but also through touch. Touch is a basic need we have as humans. In that sense, doing the exercises with a partner is also helping you to ReSYNC your brain.

For those who have trouble standing or who have a limited range of motion, I also include five exercises that work multiple muscle groups while you are seated.

With the ReSYNC Method, your muscle mass becomes lean and long. You will look more like an athlete than a body builder, and you will be preparing your body to become the best possible athlete you can be.

Reboot Your Nutritional Health with the ReSYNC Diet Plan

The word *diet* actually has two meanings. Most people think of a diet as a strict weight-loss plan. But the true meaning of the word is the totality of everything you eat. I don't believe in rigid weight-loss diets. I believe in a lifelong, healthy food plan. That said, if your nutrition is less than optimal—if, for example, you've been eating too much saturated fat or starchy carbohydrates, too little lean protein, or simply too much food—you're going to feel like what you've been eating: fat, stodgy, and heavy. You won't have the energy or the motivation to complete the exercise program or even to implement the mental and spiritual aspects of the ReSYNC plan.

Think of the ReSYNC diet as a twenty-eight-day plan to get rid of all the unhealthy stuff you may have been storing in your body and replace it with fresh and health-promoting nutrients that will get you feeling energized, clear-headed, and better about yourself virtually from day one.

I give you plenty of choices, but every option is carefully selected and researched. I'll be giving you lists of specific foods to choose from at every meal every day. Yes, the first week will be the most restrictive, because that's when you need to cleanse your system the most. But even during the first week, there will be choices you'll enjoy that will become part of your "diet" for the rest of your life. Each week the list gets longer and you get healthier as you get with the program. At the end of the twenty-eight days, you'll have a long list of foods that will allow you to maintain everything you've accomplished using the ReSYNC Method for the rest of your life.

ReSYNC Your Brain Power

As I keep saying, the ReSYNC Method is a total synergistic approach to health and well-being. I believe that brain fitness is as important to your overall fitness as diet and exercise. As your body becomes fitter, so will your brain. Physical fitness won't necessarily change your IQ, but it will allow your brain to function at its highest level. You will be more effective mentally and more focused on achieving whatever you want in life.

We've come to accept that brain function declines as we age, but exercising the brain has been shown to reduce, and possibly prevent, the decline of cognitive abilities in older people. The old adage "Use it or lose it" certainly applies here, so part of the ReSYNC Method includes daily brain boosters that will keep your mind as fit as your body.

The other side of that coin is that eating well and staying fit will also help your brain function better and increase your feelings of calmness and contentment.[1] One explanation for these results is that your brain recognizes the start of exercise as a moment of stress. Your heart rate increases and your brain goes into fight-or-flight mode, as if you were being chased by a wild animal. To protect your brain from stress, you release a protein called *brain-derived neurotrophic factor* (BDNF), which facilitates the growth of new neurons (cells that carry messages from the brain to other parts of the body), which in turn contribute to better learning, improved memory, and higher thinking.

At the same time, endorphins, which are stress-fighting chemicals, are released in your brain and help minimize whatever discomfort you might feel while you're exercising, creating that feeling often described as the runner's high. In this way exercise not only improves brain function but also elevates your mood. When you're feeling good, you tend to think more clearly, and thus the beneficial cycle continues.

Researchers at the University of Bristol in the United Kingdom found that people reported an improvement in mood and therefore in work performance on days when they exercised as opposed to days when they did not.[2]

Exercise, however, isn't the only component of the ReSYNC Method that boosts your brain and mood. Foods can also help. In chapter 4 you'll find a list of nine foods that will keep your brain working to the max. And, of course, if you also stop eating the foods that make you feel lethargic, overloaded, and lazy, your brain and your body will be working at top speed and efficiency.

ReSYNC Your Spirituality

Joel Osteen, pastor of Lakewood Church in Houston, where I developed a fitness program for members and others who were interested, believes that by being a healthier version of yourself, you can become all that God has created you to be.

In fact, the great biblical leaders, including Moses and Jesus, encouraged their followers by word and deed to eat well, be fit, and lead a healthy life.

In 1 Corinthians 6:19, for example, the apostle Paul wrote, "What? know ye not that your body is the temple of the Holy Ghost which is in you, which ye have of God, and ye are not your own?" To me, this means that your body is a precious treasure, and you need to treat it as such.

Many of the teachings in the Bible, including love, forgiveness, kindness, peace, generosity, and mindfulness, to name a few, have a profound impact on our overall health. Also, when we take the time to nourish our minds and bodies, we not only take care of our own health but also impact those around us. If you stop to think about it, you will realize that great religious leaders lead by example—they walk the walk. You'll see many examples of this in chapter 5.

Modern scholars have also noted this relationship between the spiritual and the physical. In the journal *International Scholarly Research Notices: Psychiatry*, Harold G. Koenig of Duke University reviewed the research done between 1872 and 2010 on the ways that religion and spirituality relate to mental and physical health. He wrote that "there is both qualitative and quantitative research suggesting that [religion and spirituality] helps people to deal better with adversity, either external adversity (difficult environmental circumstances) or internal adversity (genetic predisposition or vulnerability to mental disorders)."[3]

Koenig says there are many different ways in which religion and spirituality influence mental health, but the most predominant is probably that "religion provides resources for coping with stress that may increase the frequency of positive emotions and reduce the likelihood that stress will result in emotional disorders such as depression, anxiety disorder, suicide, and substance abuse. . . . While [religion and spirituality] is not a panacea, on the balance, it is generally associated with greater well-being, improved coping with stress, and better mental health."[4] And, he says, there is a great deal of evidence that better mental health also relates to better physical health. He concludes, "[Religion and spirituality] involvement should have a favorable impact on a host of physical diseases and the response of those diseases to treatment."[5]

Additionally, in a 2016 study of 74,534 women by Shanshan Li at the Chan School of Public Health in Boston, those who reported "frequent attendance at religious services" had a "significantly lower risk of all-cause, cardiovascular, and cancer mortality" than those who did not attend religious services. Based on these findings, the authors concluded, "Religion and spirituality may be an underappreciated resource that physicians could explore with their patients, as appropriate."[6]

Not only has research shown that spirituality increases overall health, but amazingly, spiritual practice also can change the brain itself. In a relatively small study of 103 adults by Lisa Miller and her colleagues at the Spirituality Mind Body Institute at Columbia University, brain MRIs showed thicker cortices in those who placed a high importance on religion or spirituality than those who did not, and Miller stated that "a relatively thicker cortex in these regions could potentially account for the protection against depression that religion or spirituality seem to afford."[7] Increasing spirituality may create physical changes in the brain that guard against depression and lead to a more peaceful and fulfilling life.

As with every other aspect of the ReSYNC Method, increasing spirituality works two ways. The more you nurture your spiritual self, the fitter you will be both mentally and physically. And the more physically fit and mentally healthy you are, the more your spirit will flourish. Many people experience a closer relationship with God. As you will see, this has, in fact, been my own experience working with the members of Lakewood Church.

Get Ready to ReSYNC Your Life

By the time you reach the end of this book, you will have all the tools you need to live better, longer, smarter, and healthier and to influence those around you to do the same. If there's one thing I've learned from working with religious and spiritual groups, it's that effort and enthusiasm are contagious. Each person's success, no matter how great or small, helps lift and inspire another to try harder and do the same. That is why, by adopting and implementing the components of the ReSYNC Method, each one of you will be helping me to fulfill my mission.

Now, it's time to get started.

CHAPTER 2

ReSYNC Your Body:
Twenty-Eight Days to Strong

Back in the days when our primitive ancestors were hunters and gatherers, their survival was based on being strong and having the ability to run, jump, climb, squat, lift, carry, throw, and catch. Since the dawn of civilization, however, our lives have been improving while our fitness, as a whole, has been declining. The more our appliances, machines, and convenience products do our work for us, the more we have to make a conscious effort to maintain or increase the strength and flexibility we once developed naturally as we went about our lives. Fitness has become an industry rather than a necessity for survival.

Fitness as a multimillion-dollar industry may be largely an invention of the twentieth century, but the importance of being physically fit as a component of overall health has been recognized for centuries. In 1553 a Spanish doctor named Cristobal Mendez wrote *El Libro del Ejercicio Corporal y de Sus*

Provechos (*The Book of Exercise and Its Advantages*), the first book to specifically address the benefits of physical exercise. Not long after that, in 1569, the Italian physician Girolamo Mercuriale published *De Arte Gymnastica* (*The Art of Gymnastics*), which was based on the ancient Greek and Roman approaches to diet and exercise and the principles of physical therapy, and is considered to be the first book on sports medicine. Since that time, hundreds if not thousands of books have been written, and schools have opened to educate people about the importance of physical fitness.

In fact, several recent studies have shown that being fit is more important for overall health than being lean.[1] That said, of course, if you exercise regularly, you are also much less likely to be overweight. By following the ReSYNC Method's plans for a healthy body through exercise and food plans, you will become both stronger and leaner quickly and for the rest of your life. The more physically fit you are as you age, the more likely you will be to retain mental acuity;[2] and the fitter you are at midlife, the less likely you will be to develop chronic diseases later on.[3]

There's no time like the present to get started.

The ReSYNC Exercise Plan Explained

The plan that I developed and that has proved successful for thousands of people is based on a combination of calisthenics and isometric strength training, using gravity and your own body's resistance to create muscle tension.

You may not have heard the term *calisthenics* in a while, and you may associate it with jumping up and down and clapping your hands over your head (which is actually a pretty good form of exercise). Calisthenics, however, is a form of exercise that involves simple movements using the weight of your own body to create resistance and build muscle while also increasing your heart rate to improve cardiovascular fitness. My program will allow you to build muscle while at the same time increasing your strength, flexibility, and endurance. Instead of isolating specific muscles or muscle groups the way working out on an exercise machine does, these exercises use multiple muscle groups simultaneously, as do most tasks of daily life.

Because aerobics, such as walking, running, or biking do not generally involve any form of resistance, you can continue doing them for relatively long periods of time. The beauty of the ReSYNC Method is that because it involves resistance, exercising multiple muscles, and increasing your heart rate all at the same time, you will accomplish much more in much less time—and all without ever having to go to a gym. In fact, as you will see, the entry-level exercise program takes only ten minutes.

Before You Begin

There are two levels of the ReSYNC Method exercise plan, each with two parts. Level 1, Part 1, as I said, takes just ten minutes. Level 1, Part 2, takes twenty-five minutes, including a five-minute rest period. Level 2, Part 1, takes the same amount of time but involves more advanced exercises, while Level 2, Part 2, takes forty minutes plus a five-minute rest period.

Before you begin you need to determine your current level of fitness. Most people begin at Level 1, so don't think that you need to be a hero and start out at a higher level. Doing that will only put you at risk for injury and ultimately set you back instead of moving you forward. So when you answer the five questions in the self-assessment test that follows, be totally honest about how you score.

The ReSYNC Method Self-Assessment Test

Push-Up Test. How many push-ups can you do right now? Men should do standard push-ups; women may prefer to do knee push-ups. I can do _____ push-ups.

Crunch Test. Lie on the floor on your back, knees bent, feet flat on the floor, hands lightly touching your ears. Lift your shoulder blades off the floor, and then lie back down. How many can you do? I can do _____ crunches.

Squat Test. Stand with your feet shoulder-width apart. Bend your knees and send your rear-end back as if you were about to sit in a chair. Squat, raising your arms straight out in front of you, until your thighs are almost parallel to the floor. Don't go too quickly—take at least three seconds to lower yourself. Come back up slowly as you lower your arms. Take at least two seconds to rise back up. Repeat. How many squats can you do? I can do _____ squats.

Balance Test. Stand up straight, about three feet from a wall or counter. Look at a clock or watch with a second hand. Raise your right foot off the floor. How many seconds can you stand on one foot before you have to lower it or grab onto something? Write it down. Now do the same thing with the other foot. Then do it one more time on each foot, and average all four scores. I can balance on one foot for an average of _____ seconds.

Cardio Test. For this test, you will need a kitchen timer, a stopwatch, or a heart-rate monitor. Set it for one minute. Do jumping jacks vigorously until the minute is up, and immediately check your heart rate, either with the monitor or by measuring your pulse for fifteen seconds and multiplying that number by four. After one minute of jumping jacks, my heart rate is _____ beats per minute.

Now score yourself for each exercise to determine the ReSYNC fitness level at which you should begin. Circle the level next to the score that more closely matches your actual numbers.

Push-Up Score:

20 or fewer: Level 1

More than 20: Level 2

Crunch Score:

50 or fewer: Level 1

More than 50: Level 2

Squat Score:

25 or fewer: Level 1

More than 25: Level 2

Balance Score:

Less than 10 seconds: Level 1

More than 10 seconds: Level 2

Cardio Score:

Heart rate 110 beats per minute or higher: Level 1

Heart rate 110 beats per minute or lower: Level 2

Now count the number of times your scores are paired with Level 1 and with Level 2. The level at which you score most often—for three or more out of the five exercises—is the level at which you should start. For example, if you scored Level 2 on two tests but Level 1 on three tests, start with Level 1. If you have any doubt at all about where you should begin, even if you test at Level 2 on four out of the five tests, you would be wise to begin at Level 1.

Level 1 provides a vigorous workout for most people, and only those who are already very fit will feel comfortable starting at Level 2. You can always move up if Level 1 proves to be too easy, but starting at too high a level could cause you to injure yourself.

You will be amazed at how quickly you see results. Within the first week, you will notice increased strength, energy, and firming. And when you combine the fitness plan with the diet plan in the next chapter, you will quickly begin dropping excess pounds and replacing fat with muscle.

The Ten Nutrients You Need When You're Working Out

When you start working out regularly, you need to be sure you're getting enough of the specific nutrients that are likely to be depleted as you become more active. Try incorporating the foods listed here in your diet to ensure against nutrient loss:

Vitamin B: tuna, black beans, lentils, and peanuts
Calcium: milk, yogurt, leafy greens, beans, and fortified cereals
Vitamin C: oranges, strawberries, bell peppers, and kale
Vitamin D: milk, salmon, trout, and egg yolks
Vitamin E: sunflower seeds, almonds, and peanut butter
Iron: beef, eggs, spinach, broccoli, and fortified cereals
Magnesium: leafy greens, almonds, halibut, and quinoa
Potassium: sweet potatoes, bananas, avocados, and tuna
Sodium: pretzels and salted nuts
Zinc: red meat, chickpeas, pumpkin seeds, and quinoa

The ReSYNC Exercise Plan

Work through the exercises below on four days of the week. Choose two other days to do thirty minutes of some type of cardio, such as walking, jogging, biking, or working out on an elliptical trainer or treadmill. Choose one day for rest. Your week might look like this:

Monday: ReSYNC Level 1:1
Tuesday: Walking
Wednesday: ReSYNC Level 1:1
Thursday: ReSYNC Level 1:1
Friday: Biking
Saturday: ReSYNC Level 1:1
Sunday: Rest Day

Level 1:1—Ten-Minute Workout

You will be doing a one-minute warm-up and actively resting for one minute between the exercises. Stay at this level for as long as you need to. This could be a week, a month, or even three months. As long as the workout feels strenuous, you are where you are supposed to be. When you get to the point where Level 1:1 is starting to feel easy, your muscles aren't fatigued, and your heart rate is below 130 when you finish, you can move to Level 1:2.

Warm-Up: Power Walk (1 minute). Walk while moving your arms up and down, elbows bent, in opposite directions.

Exercise 1: Tension Walk (1 minute). Stand with feet hip-width apart, and walk forward while keeping your entire body tense and pumping your arms up and down in opposite directions. It is important to keep your body tensed the entire time. Imagine you are walking through water or mud.

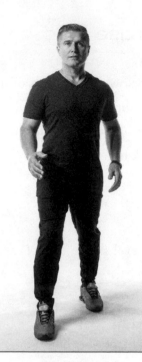

Power Walk (A)

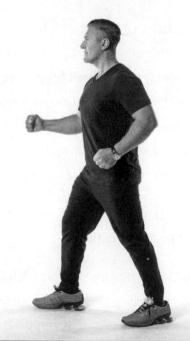

Power Walk (B)

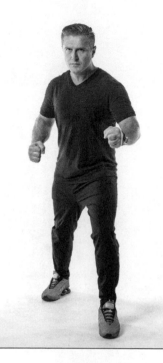

Tension Walk (A)

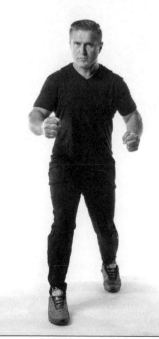

Tension Walk (B)

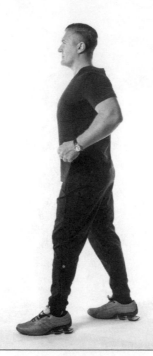

Shrug Walk (A)

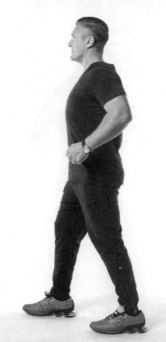

Shrug Walk (B)

Active Rest: Shrug Walk (1 minute). Walk with your shoulders raised, as if you were shrugging and stopped halfway through.

Exercise 2: Hercules Push (30 seconds on each leg). Find some empty wall space (or, if you're outside, a tree). Face the wall and put one leg forward so that you have a stable pushing position. Place your palms flat on the wall, hands 5 inches apart and elbows slightly bent. Tighten your entire body, and push the wall as hard as you can, as if you would like to move it. Hold that position for 30 seconds; then switch legs.

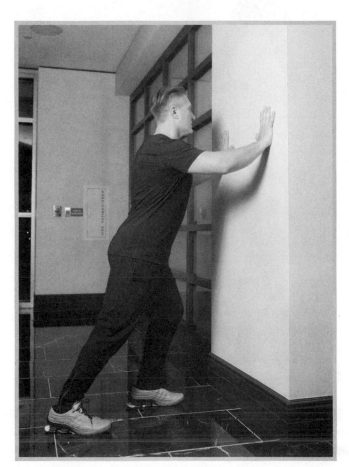

Hercules Push

Active Rest: Frankenstein Walk (1 minute). Walk with your arms extended in front of your chest, elbows slightly bent.

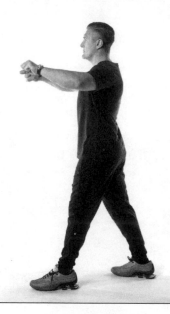

Frankenstein Walk (A)

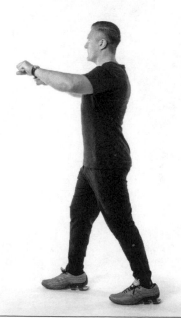

Frankenstein Walk (B)

Exercise 3: Achilles Tension Squat (1 minute). Stand with the feet shoulder-width apart. Make your hands into fists, tense your arms, and raise them in front of you, elbows slightly bent. Tighten your abdominal muscles, and slowly start to squat by bending your hips and knees until your thighs are at least parallel to the floor. (If bending that deep is too difficult at first, just bend as far as you can.) Make sure to keep your feet flat on the floor and your knees no farther forward than your toes. Press down on your heels as you return to a standing position. Do at least 20 reps in 1 minute.

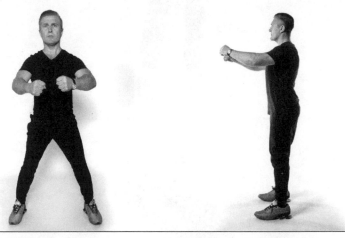

Achilles Tension Squat (A)

Achilles Tension Squat (B)

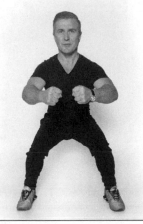

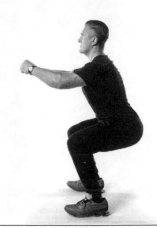

Achilles Tension Squat (C)

Achilles Tension Squat (D)

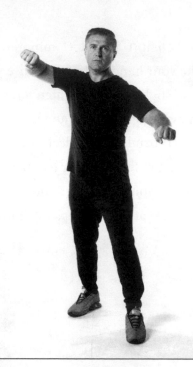

Penguin Walk (A)

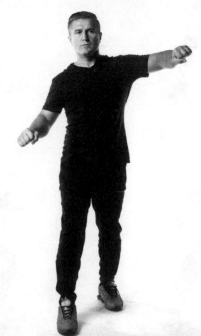

Penguin Walk (B)

Active Rest: Penguin Walk (1 minute). Walk with elbows bent, arms held away from your body, one arm slightly higher than the other.

Exercise 4: Ares Side Push (30 seconds on each side). Stand with the left side of your body touching a wall. Bend your knees 2 inches, and lean your left shoulder and arm against the wall. Tighten your entire body, and push the wall as hard as you can. Hold for 30 seconds, and switch sides.

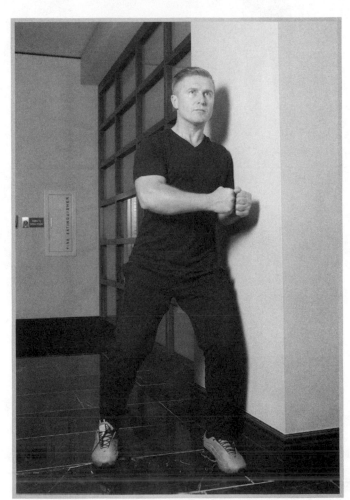

Ares Side Push

Active Rest: Superman Walk (1 minute). Walk with your arms extended over your head and slightly in front of you.

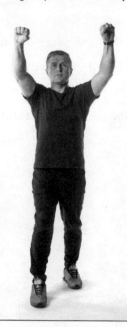

Superman Walk (A)

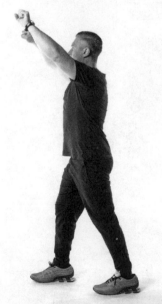

Superman Walk (B)

Exercise 5: Sisyphus Push (30 seconds on each side). Stand with your feet hip-width apart. Step forward on your left leg, and slowly lower your body until your left thigh is parallel to the floor. (If bending that deeply is too difficult at first, just bend your knee as much as you can.) As you do this, raise your arms bending your elbows until your hands are just in front of your chest. Tighten your muscles, and as you straighten your left knee, push your arms out forward as if you were pushing something away from you. (Change legs after 30 seconds.)

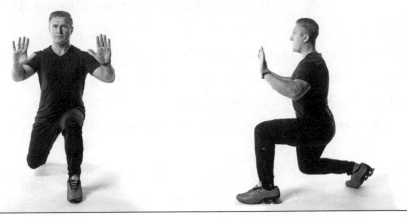

Sisyphus Push (A)

Sisyphus Push (B)

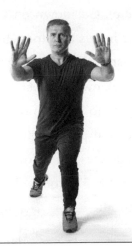

Sisyphus Push (C)

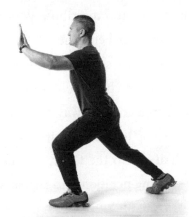

Sisyphus Push (D)

Level 1:2—Twenty-Minute Workout and Five-Minute Rest Period

For Level 1:2, simply do Level 1:1 twice with 5 minutes of rest in between. This should take a total of 25 minutes. When you get to the point where you can do Level 1:2 in 25 minutes, it feels easy, your muscles are not fatigued, and your heart rate is not above 130 when you have completed the workout, you are ready for Level 2:1.

Level 2:1—Twenty-Minute Workout and Five-Minute Rest Period

Combine the five exercises from Level 1:1 with the five described in the following section so that you are doing a total of ten exercises with active resting in between. The active resting for Level 2 involves running in place instead of walking. Take a 5-minute rest after the first five exercises.

Warm Up: Power Run (1 minute). Run in place while moving your arms up and down, elbows bent, in opposite directions.

Exercise 1: Push-Up-and-a-Half (1 minute). Get down on the floor, facing down, and distribute your weight on your hands and toes (beginners can be on their bent knees). Keeping your body straight, your feet together, and your hands shoulder-width apart, bend your elbows to lower your body, bringing your chest close to the floor. (Make sure to keep your elbows no more than 3 inches away from your body.) Hold that position for 1 second; then push up to your starting position. Bend your elbows again, lowering your body halfway to the floor, and hold that position for 5 seconds. Push up to your starting position and repeat. Do this for 1 minute.

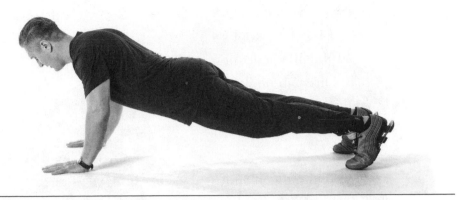

Push-Up-and-a-Half (A)

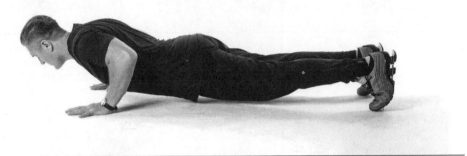

Push-Up-and-a-Half (B)

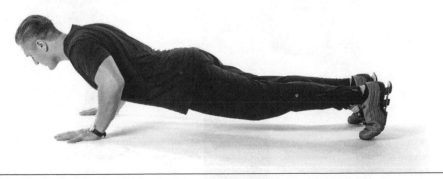

Push-Up-and-a-Half (C)

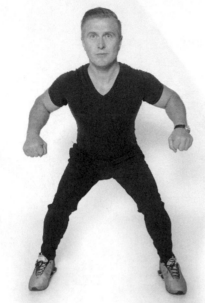
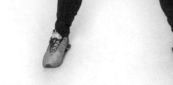

Aphrodite Squat (A)

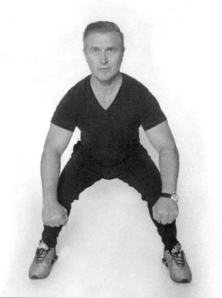

Aphrodite Squat (B)

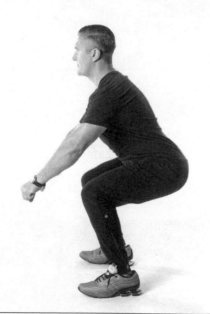

Aphrodite Squat (C)

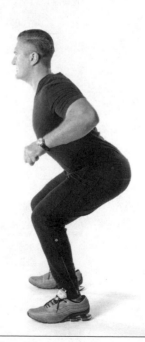

Aphrodite Squat (D)

Active Rest: Shrug Run (1 minute). Run in place, pumping your knees high, with your shoulders raised as if you were shrugging and stopped halfway through.

Exercise 2: Aphrodite Squat (1 minute). Standing with your feet shoulder-width apart, squat down 5 to 6 inches (your thighs should never be parallel to the floor). Bend forward slightly at the hips, arms down, hands shoulder-width apart. Tense your body, bend your elbows, and slowly lift your hands toward the sides of your chest while at the same time straightening your legs 2 to 3 inches, keeping your knees bent at all times. Hold for 1 second; then slowly return to your starting position. Repeat for a total of 1 minute.

Active Rest: Frankenstein Run (1 minute). Run in place, pumping your knees high, with your arms extended in front of your chest, elbows slightly bent (see Frankenstein Walk for reference).

Exercise 3: Pharaoh Dance (1 minute). Stand with your feet shoulder-width apart. Make your hands into fists, bend your arms at the elbow, and raise them to either side of your body. Keeping your arms in that position, tense your body, and bend your knees until your thighs are parallel to the floor. Keeping your body tensed, raise yourself 5 to 6 inches from the full squat, and raise your arms above your shoulders. Go back into the squat, and return your arms to the starting position. Make sure to keep your arms tensed as if you are holding heavy weights. If you would like to make the exercise more challenging, hold a pair of 5-to 15-pound dumbbells, depending on your own size and strength. Start with 5 pounds, and if that's too easy, increase the weight.

Active Rest: Penguin Run (1 minute). Run in place, pumping your knees high, elbows bent, arms held away from your body, one slightly higher than the other (see photos of Penguin Walk for reference).

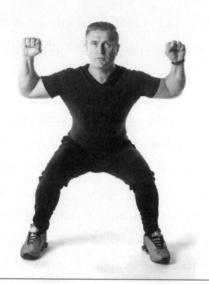

Pharaoh Dance (A)

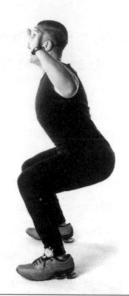

Pharaoh Dance (B)

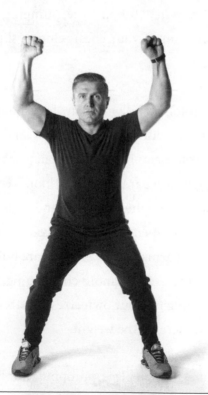

Pharaoh Dance (C)

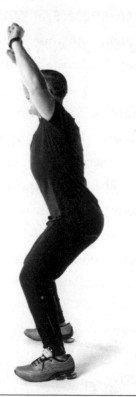

Pharaoh Dance (D)

Exercise 4: Samson Pose (30 seconds on each side). Find the end of a wall. Stand next to the wall with one leg forward, knees bent. Grab the sides of the wall with both hands, keeping your elbows slightly bent. Tighten your entire body, and with all your strength pull on the wall as if you wanted to move it. Make sure to keep your body tensed and to keep pulling with all your strength for 30 seconds; then switch sides and repeat for another 30 seconds.

Active Rest: Superman Run (1 minute). Run in place, pumping your knees high, with your arms extended over your head and slightly in front of you (see photos of Superman Walk for reference).

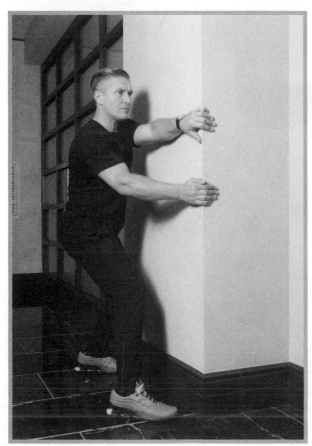

Samson Pose

Exercise 5: Atlas Pose (30 seconds on each side). Stand with your feet shoulder-width apart. Move one leg forward, and bend your knee until your thigh is parallel to the floor. Bend your arms, elbows out to your sides, forearms straight up so that your hands are level with your ears. Keeping your arms tense and stationary, press up with your legs and return to your starting position. Hold for 1 second and repeat. After 30 seconds, switch legs. You should be able to do a total of 40 lunges—20 on each side—in 1 minute.

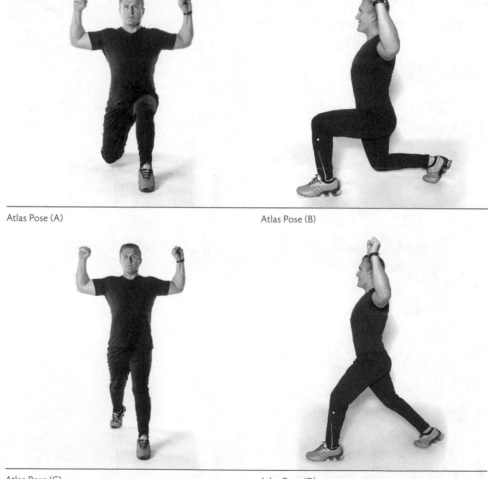

Atlas Pose (A)

Atlas Pose (B)

Atlas Pose (C)

Atlas Pose (D)

Exercises 6–10: Do the five exercises and active rest movements from Level 1:1, making sure to run rather than walk during the active rests.

Level 2:2—Forty-Minute Workout and Five-Minute Rest Period

For Level 2:2, do all the exercises for Level 2:1 twice, with a 5-minute rest period in between. You can do stretches during your rest.

Partner Exercises

Partner exercises not only provide a dynamic workout with periods of active resting but also provide a way to ReSYNC with friends and family as you ReSYNC yourself.

Level 1:1—Ten-Minute Partner Workout

Warm Up: Power Walk (1 minute). See page 28. Walk while moving your arms up and down, elbows bent, in opposite directions. Do this either facing your partner or side by side facing a mirror.

Partner Exercise 1: Compromise (1 minute). Stand facing your partner. Both partners: Move your right leg one step back, and extend your right arm straight forward, making a fist. Bend your left elbow, and keep your left hand open. Each partner should push his or her fist into the partner's open hand. Making sure that your hands never separate, push back and forth, right-left, right-left, while your partner resists the push. Just as in a relationship, you need to find a balance. It's not about who is stronger; it is about synchronizing your bodies. Do this for 1 minute.

Active Rest: Shrug Walk (1 Minute). See page 30. Walk with your shoulders raised, as if you were shrugging and stopped halfway through. Do this either facing your partner or side by side facing a mirror.

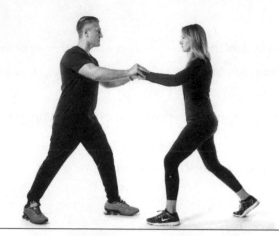

Compromiseex (A)

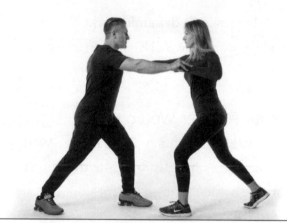

Compromise (B)

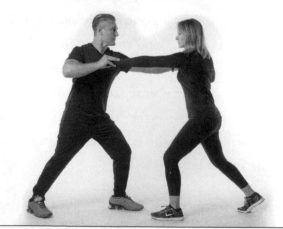

Compromise (C)

Partner Exercise 2: Synchronize (1 minute). Facing each other, hold hands, bend your knees, and squat. Make sure your knees don't go past your toes. Now, alternating arms, start pulling and resisting. While partner A pulls with one arm, partner B resists, and vice versa. This is not about who is stronger but about listening and feeling how much resistance your partner needs while you both get a good workout. Do this for 1 minute.

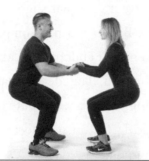

Synchronize (A)

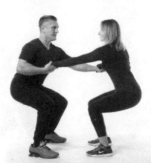

Synchronize (B)

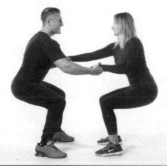

Synchronize (B)

Active Rest: Frankenstein Walk (1 minute). See page 32. Walk with your arms extended in front of your chest, elbows slightly bent. Do this either facing your partner or side by side facing a mirror.

Partner Exercise 3: Support (1 minute). Stand with partner A in front and partner B in back. Partner B: Step back with one leg, and place your hands on partner A's upper back. Partner A: Squat slightly while leaning your back into partner B's hands. Partner B: Start pushing on partner A's back and walking forward. Partner A: Tighten your abdominals, and while resisting partner B's push, start taking steps forward. The idea is that you give enough resistance so that the person pushing you can feel it but you keep walking forward. Do not lean back. Keep walking for 30 seconds; then switch roles. This is about giving and accepting support.

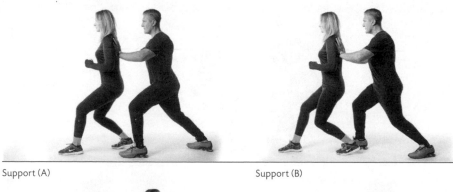

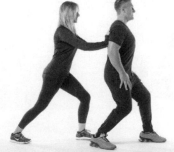

Support (A)

Support (B)

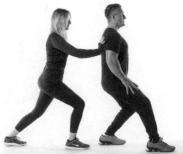

Support (C)

Support (D)

Active Rest: Penguin Walk (1 minute). See page 34. Walk with elbows bent, arms held away from your body, one arm slightly higher than the other. Do this either facing your partner or side by side facing a mirror.

Partner Exercise 4: Trust (1 minute). Stand facing your partner. Extend your arms forward. Partner A: Make your hands into fists, and position them in Partner B's hands. Make sure your elbows are slightly bent. Take a step forward, pushing partner B backward. Partner B: Resist the push as you slowly take a step back. Trust your partner to lead you. Keep walking for 30 seconds; then switch roles.

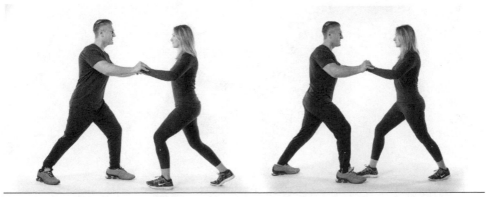

Trust (A)   Trust (B)

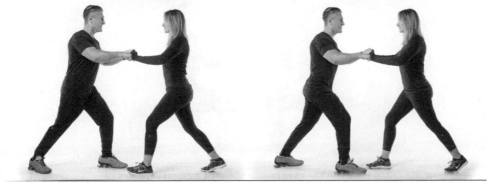

Trust (C)   Trust (D)

Active Rest: Superman Walk (1 minute). See page 36. Walk with your arms extended over your head and slightly in front of you. Do this either facing your partner or side by side facing a mirror.

Partner Exercise 5: Harmony (1 minute). Facing each other, hold hands and bend your knees until your thighs are parallel to the floor. Make sure your elbows are slightly bent. While staying in the squat position, keeping your arms still and in the starting position, partner A slowly pulls on partner B's hands so there is tension at all times. Find the harmony between you and your partner to balance the pull and resistance. Partner A keeps pulling for 30 seconds while partner B keeps resisting. Switch roles after 30 seconds.

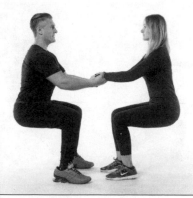

Harmony (A)

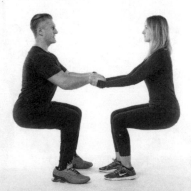

Harmony (B)

Level 1:2 Partner Workout—Twenty Minutes and Five-Minute Rest Period

If you would like to make it more difficult but are not ready to move on to Level 2, simply rest for 5 minutes after completing Level 1:1, and repeat the workout with your partner.

Level 2:1 Partner Workout—Twenty Minutes

Repeat Level 1:1, doing each exercise for a total of 2 minutes. If you are switching roles in the exercise, change after 1 minute instead of 30 seconds.

Level 2:2 Partner Workout—Forty Minutes and Five-Minute Rest Period

Repeat Level 2:1 with a 5-minute rest period in between.

Seated Exercises

You can benefit from the ReSYNC Method workout even while you are seated. The following exercises are designed to accommodate anyone who is not able to do standing or walking exercises.

Exercise 1: Upper-Body Tense. While seated in a straight-backed chair, place your feet flat on the floor and hip-width apart. Tighten your abdominal muscles. Make fists with both hands, and bring your arms in front of you, holding them 2 to 3 inches above your legs. Tighten the muscles in your arms, chest, and shoulders as hard as you can, and hold for 10 to 30 seconds. Take a 30-second break and repeat 4 times.

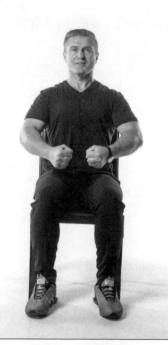

Upper Body Tense (A)

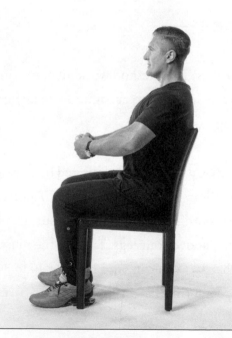

Upper Body Tense (B)

Exercise 2: Tension Shoulder Press. While seated in a straight-backed chair, place your feet flat on the floor and hip-width apart. Tighten your abdominal muscles. Make fists with both hands. Hold your arms out to your sides at shoulder height, and bend your elbows to raise your upper arms beside your head. Tighten your arm muscles, and imagine that you are holding a 100-pound weight in each hand. Now raise those weights above your head by extending your arms. Keeping your muscles tense, slowly bring your arms down to the starting position. Repeat 10 times, take a 30-second break, and do 3 more sets of 10. (If you have limited range of motion or extending your arms above your head is too difficult, simply keep your hands in the starting position, tighten your arm muscles as hard as you can, and hold that position for 10 to 30 seconds.)

Exercise 3: Tension Chest Press-Pull. Sit in a straight-backed chair with your feet flat on the floor and hip-width apart. Tighten your abdominal muscles. Make fists with both hands, lift your arms to shoulder height, and bend your elbows so that your hands are facing forward at shoulder height. Now imagine that you have to push a 300-pound weight forward. Tense your chest and arm muscles and slowly extend your arms straight out in front of you, pushing the weight away. Hold that position for 1 second, and slowly pull the weight back to your original position. Repeat 10 times. The key is to maintain the tension in your arms and chest at all times while pushing and pulling. Do 4 sets with a 30-second break between each one. (If you have limited range of motion, hold your arms in the starting position for 10 to 30 seconds with your muscles tensed as hard as you can.)

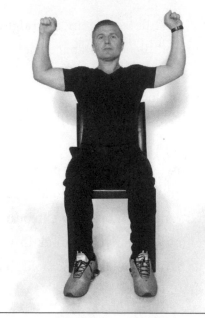

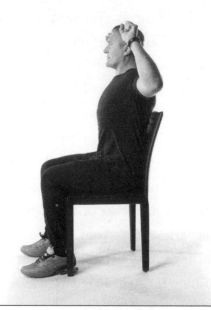

Tension Shoulder Press (A)

Tension Shoulder Press (B)

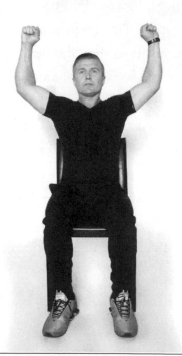

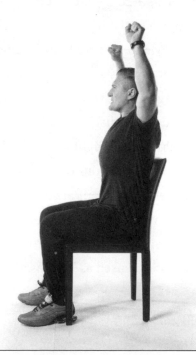

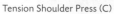

Tension Shoulder Press (C)

Tension Shoulder Press (D)

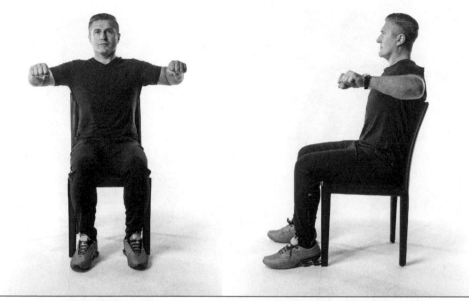

Tension Chest Press-Pull (A)

Tension Chest Press-Pull (B)

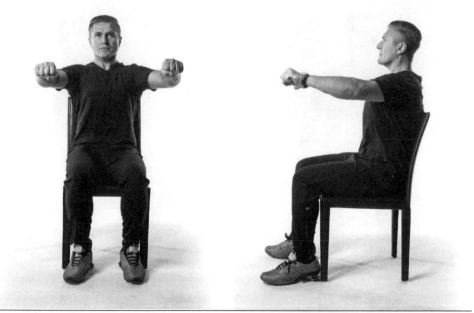

Tension Chest Press-Pull (C)

Tension Chest Press-Pull (D)

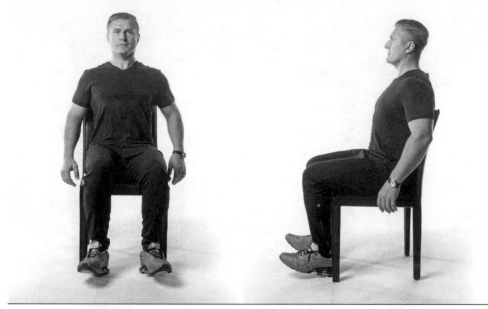

Leg Tension (A)   Leg Tension (B)

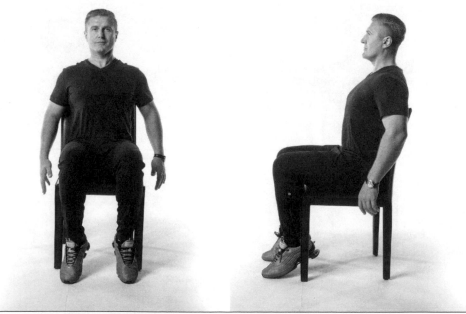

Leg Tension (C)   Leg Tension (D)

Exercise 4: Leg Tension. Sit in a straight-backed chair with your feet flat on the floor and hip-width apart. Lift your toes up while keeping your heels on the floor. Tighten your abdominal muscles, your glutes, and your leg muscles while pushing down with your heels. Hold that position for 30 seconds. Take a 30-second break. Now raise your heels and push down with your toes while still holding your abdominals, glutes, and legs as tight as possible. Hold that position for 30 seconds. Repeat 4 times. (If you have limited range of motion, keep your feet flat on the floor while tensing the muscles in your lower body as much as you can. Hold the tension for 30 seconds.)

Exercise 5: Full Body Tension. Sitting in a straight-backed chair with feet hip-width apart, raise your heels while keeping your toes on the floor. Tighten your abdominal muscles as hard as you can. Make your hands into fists, and allow your arms to hang down on either side of your body. Now tighten all the muscles in your body, and imagine you are holding a 30-pound weight in each hand. Slowly bend your arms close to your body so that your forearms are parallel to the floor and your fists are facing each other. With your muscles still tensed, hold that position for 1 second. Then, focusing on your triceps and still resisting those 30-pound weights, slowly bring your arms back to the starting position. Make sure that you keep all the muscles throughout your body tensed during the entire exercise. Repeat 10 times. Do 4 sets with a 30-second break between each set. (If you have limited range of motion, simply tighten all the muscles in your body without lifting your arms, and hold the tension for 30 seconds. Repeat 4 times with 30-second breaks.)

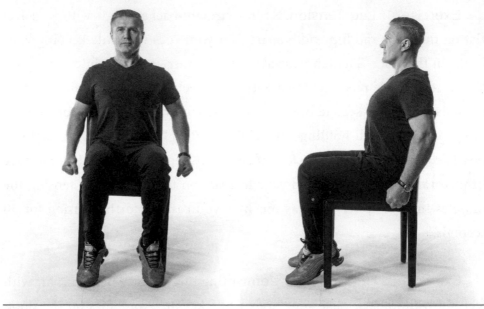

Full Body Tension (A)   Full Body Tension (B)

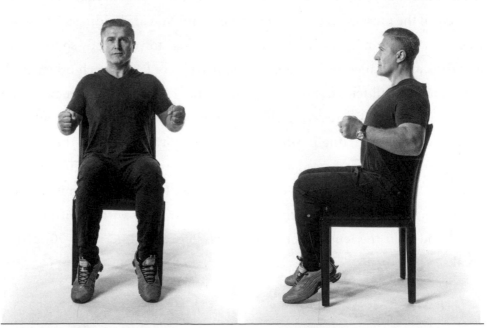

Full Body Tension (C)   Full Body Tension (D)

CHAPTER THREE

ReSYNC Your Diet: Twenty-Eight Days to Lean and Healthy

Let food be thy medicine, and medicine be thy food.
—HIPPOCRATES, THE FATHER OF MODERN MEDICINE (C. 460-C. 375 BC)

Since ancient times, humans have been seeking to determine how the foods we eat impact our health and how food can be used to treat or even eradicate various illnesses. The first written account of a disease that appears to be what we now call scurvy (caused by a deficiency in vitamin C) is in the Ebers Papyrus, which dates to about 1500 BC in Egypt. The writer not only described the disease but also recommended that victims be treated with onions, which are a common source of vitamin C.[1] And even today, particularly in developing countries, herbal cures are still often the primary source of "medical treatment" for thousands of people.

Modern medicine, of course, has saved millions of lives, and I would never suggest that anyone who is truly ill should not take advantage of everything medicine has to offer. What I do say, however, is that if you follow a nutritious diet, you are likely to avoid many of the health problems that would otherwise send you to the doctor and potentially shorten your life. By the way, it appears that Hippocrates himself lived to be approximately eighty-five years old—an extraordinary age for his time.

Water, Life's Most Essential Ingredient

Why do you think NASA scientists were so excited when they discovered signs of water on Mars? Because, throughout history, wherever we've found water, we've discovered some form of life. If there is no water, there can be no life.

The average adult human body is composed of 50 to 65 percent water. Without water we would shrivel up and die, just like a flower. Therefore, simply from a cosmetic point of view, if all you want is radiant, healthy-looking skin, you should be sure to drink plenty of water. But, of course, there's much more to it than that.

Water promotes weight loss not only by making you feel fuller longer so that you are likely to eat less[2] but also by boosting your metabolism. A study by Michael Boschmann published in the *Journal of Clinical Endocrinology and Metabolism* showed that drinking 500 milliliters (approximately 17 ounces) of water increased metabolic rate by 30 percent.[3]

Water also improves kidney function so that you digest and eliminate foods—as well as toxins—from your body more efficiently.[4]

When your cells, including your muscle cells, are not properly hydrated, they can't function properly, which is why it's particularly important that you drink water when you exercise.[5]

Clean Water Is Key to a Healthy Life

For millennia people have recognized the need for clean drinking water. The Romans built nine massive aqueducts to deliver fresh water across Italy. While poor by our standards, it was the cleanest water available until the late 1800s, when Louis Pasteur proved that microbes in water could transmit disease. But it wasn't until 1974 that the US Congress passed the Safe Drinking Water Act to ensure that all Americans had access to clean water. In developing countries throughout the world, access to clean drinking water is still a major problem.

Studies have also shown that even mild dehydration causes changes in mood and brain function in both men and women. In one study, conducted by Matthew S. Ganio of the Texas Health Presbyterian Hospital in Dallas and published in the *British Journal of Nutrition*, the researchers concluded that "mild dehydration . . . in men, induced adverse changes in vigilance and working memory, and increased tension/anxiety and fatigue."[6] But dehydration is a problem for women too. A study by Lawrence E. Armstrong at the University of Connecticut and published in the *Journal of Nutrition*, found that "degraded mood, increased perception of task difficulty, lower concentration, and headache symptoms resulted from 1.36% dehydration in females."[7]

The USDA recommends that adult men get 3.7 liters (about one gallon) and women 2.7 liters (about three-fourths of a gallon) of water *from all sources* (including foods and other beverages) in a day.[8] But I want you to drink even more—ideally a gallon a day *in addition to* whatever water you consume from other sources.

In fact, if I had only one piece of advice to give you, it would be to drink plenty of water.

Why Put Lemon or Lime in Your Water?

Putting a squeeze of fresh lemon or lime in your water has many benefits beyond those of the water itself:

- Because citrus juice is similar to the digestive secretions found naturally in your body, it helps to improve digestion.
- It contains antioxidants that help flush free radicals from your body.
- It allows your body to absorb more iron, which, in turn, boosts your immune system.
- It contains vitamin C, which promotes healthy bones and teeth, is good for your skin, and improves eyesight.
- It acts as a natural diuretic, which helps flush toxins from your body.

ReSYNC Your Digestive System

If you're used to eating heavy, fatty, sugary, starchy foods, your digestive system is probably exhausted. Even when you're sleeping, your digestive system is still working to process all that food you've been eating. In fact, I would say that we in America have a chronic digestive problem that is impacting our overall health. A tired digestive system cannot absorb and metabolize nutrients properly. Food that is not properly digested remains in your body, where it can ultimately create toxic byproducts that lead to serious gastrointestinal problems including colitis and irritable bowel syndrome.

A study by the National Food Institute, Technical University of Denmark, found "that the longer food takes to pass through the colon, the more harmful bacterial degradation products are produced."[9]

That's why, as you will see, the first seven days of the ReSYNC diet plan are the most restrictive. By eating good, clean food and not overeating, you will allow your digestive system to get some much-needed rest so that it starts to function at its fullest potential.

In addition to being affected by what we eat, our digestive system is also impacted by *how* we eat. Because we lead such busy lives, too many of us these days are eating on the go or at our desks while we're doing something else. When we do that, we're also usually eating too fast and often not even tasting the food.

It takes about twenty minutes for the message "you're full" to be delivered from your gut to your brain. So if you're eating too fast, chances are you're also eating well beyond the point where you're actually full. Take twenty minutes out of your day to slow down and eat your food, paying attention to how it looks, how it smells, and how it tastes. Not only your digestive system but also your waistline will thank you for it. [10]

The Difference Between Digestion and Metabolism

Digestion refers to how your body processes the food you eat and eliminates waste products. Metabolism refers to the way your body uses (or burns) the energy (that is, calories) you have absorbed during the digestive process. Both can be either fast or slow, but they are not the same thing.[11]

Eat Good Protein

Every single cell in your body contains protein. It is essential for building and maintaining cellular structure. The muscles, hormones, enzymes, and antibodies in your body are all made of protein, and if you don't get enough of it, eventually your organs will break down and cease to function.

Protein also works to keep you energized by raising levels of tyrosine, an amino acid that signals the brain to manufacture norepinephrine and dopamine, which help regulate mood.

Amino acids are the building blocks of protein. Our bodies are able to manufacture most types of amino acids, but a few, called essential amino acids, including omega-3 and omega-6, must be obtained from food sources. Individual animal sources of protein (called complete proteins) generally include all the essential amino acids, while plant sources often need to be eaten in combination, because individually they may lack one or more of the essential amino acids.

No Need to Fear Eating Eggs

For a long time we've been told to avoid eating whole eggs because the yolks contain a lot of cholesterol. Recent studies, however, have shown that the cholesterol in eggs doesn't raise blood cholesterol in the majority of people and has no effect on the risk for heart disease in otherwise healthy people.[12] In fact, eggs are extremely nutritious, containing important nutrients for the brain and antioxidants that help protect your eyesight.

The problem for many people is choosing the right proteins, because many animal sources come bundled with unhealthy saturated fats. "Good" animal protein sources include fish and seafood (particularly wild salmon), skinless white-meat poultry, lean meats, eggs, and Greek yogurt.

Plant sources of protein include nuts, beans, and seeds. Quinoa is a whole grain that is the only plant source of complete protein. In addition, it contains significant amounts of important antioxidants that are found only in plant foods. For these reasons it is often considered one of the healthiest foods in the world.

If you follow the ReSYNC diet that follows, you will be getting the right amount of protein from all the right sources.

Protein for Breakfast Helps Keep You Full

A study by H. J. Leidy of the Department of Foods and Nutrition at Purdue University, published in the *British Journal of Nutrition*, has shown that eating protein for breakfast while on a restricted-calorie diet keeps you feeling fuller longer throughout the day.[13]

We Need Healthy Fats

Many of you have probably heard that fat makes you fat. And it's true that a gram of fat has more than twice as many calories as a gram of protein or carbohydrate. But that's only part of the story. You need healthy fats in order for your body—including your brain—to function. In fact, your brain is about 60 percent fat, the greatest concentration in any single organ of the healthy human body.

Fats are necessary to maintain strong and healthy cell membranes. On the most basic level, cell membranes separate the interior of each cell from the external environment and determine which substances should be allowed in or out of the cell. If the membrane detects a toxic substance, it will not allow it to enter the cell. So, as you can see, if you don't have healthy cell membranes, all kinds of bad stuff would be allowed to permeate your cells and make you sick—or, potentially, kill you.

But that doesn't mean you should eat more fat or that all fats are created equal. "Good" fats are monounsaturated and polyunsaturated and are found mainly in olive and other vegetable oils, fish, seafood, nuts, and seeds. In addition to their role in maintaining the integrity of your cells, monounsaturated fats help to raise HDL (good) cholesterol. Good fats—including omega-3 and omega-6 fatty acids—also help reduce overall cholesterol and triglyceride levels, fight inflammation on the cellular level, and lower blood pressure. In addition, omega-3s can help boost serotonin levels in the brain, improving your mood and increasing your motivation to stay away from the Double Stuf Oreos.

A study conducted by M. Micallef of the University of Newcastle in New South Wales, Australia and published in the *British Journal of Nutrition* showed that study participants with the highest blood levels of polyunsaturated fats had the lowest body mass index, hip circumference, and waist circumference, indicating that polyunsaturated fat may play a role in weight control and amounts of belly fat.[14]

"Bad" or saturated fats are the ones that clog up your arteries and increase your risk for heart disease. They are found mainly in red meat and full-fat dairy products, including cheese.

A study by Olivia I. Okereke of Brigham and Women's Hospital and Harvard Medical School, published in the *Annals of Neurology*, found that higher intakes of saturated fats were associated with worse cognitive function and verbal memory, while higher intakes of monounsaturated fats were associated with better cognitive function and verbal memory. And these results appeared to be influenced more by the specific type of fat than the total amount consumed.[15]

Trans fats are the worst of the worst. Although they begin life as liquid unsaturated fat, they are altered through a chemical process to make them solid at room temperature. Trans fats are found mainly in processed foods such as baked goods, snacks such as potato chips, and fried foods, because the fat helps keep these foods fresh longer. At the same time, it lowers good (HDL) cholesterol and raises bad (LDL) cholesterol, which is exactly the opposite of what you need to maintain heart health.

Carbs Are Not Your Enemy

As is true for both proteins and fats, there are also healthy and unhealthy carbohydrates. Unfortunately, many people think they need to avoid *all* carbohydrates to maintain a healthy weight. What they don't realize is that carbohydrates are the main source of energy for your body, including your brain. A 2008 study at Tufts University is worth noting because it shows that when people eliminated carbs to diet, they performed worse on memory tasks than people who cut calories but maintained carb intake.[16]

Essentially, if you don't eat enough carbs, your body will start to burn protein for energy, and not only is protein a less efficient source of energy, but also you need to use it for other functions—not for fuel.

So why have carbs gotten such a bad rap? People tend to associate carbohydrates with sugary or starchy foods they think of as "fattening" and don't realize that *all* plant foods (that is, anything that ever grew in the ground or on a bush or tree), including all fruits and vegetables, are carbohydrates. They aren't aware of the difference between carbs we digest quickly and those that take a longer time for our bodies to process.

Carbs that metabolize quickly include refined sugar, refined white flour (such as white bread, white rice, and white pasta), as well as cakes and cookies. All carbohydrates are metabolized as sugar (glucose), and the ones we digest quickly cause blood sugar levels to spike and over time can lead to insulin resistance and, ultimately, diabetes.

In the past century, Americans have increased their consumption of fructose, in the form of refined sugar and high-fructose corn syrup, from 15 to 75 grams per day. In Grandma's day, cakes and pastries were considered treats reserved for holidays and special occasions. Now we're eating these and other sugary sweets every day, as well as drinking huge quantities of soda, which contains high-fructose corn syrup.[17]

When blood sugar levels rise, your body automatically produces insulin, which works to remove the glucose from your blood and move it into your cells, where it can be used for energy. But when there's more glucose than you

Make Friends with the Glycemic Index

The glycemic index is a system for ranking foods on a scale of 1 to 100 based on how quickly they raise blood sugar levels. You will want to seek out carbs that are *low* on the glycemic index. Sweetness is not necessarily the key. For example, cherries have a glycemic index of 9, while strawberries come in at just 1. You can find the glycemic index for 100 foods at www.health.harvard.edu/diseases-and-conditions/glycemic_index_and_glycemic_load_for_100_foods.

need for energy, the excess gets stored as fat. And with constantly elevated blood sugar levels, your body can become resistant to insulin, meaning that diabetes is imminent.

Carbohydrates that take longer to digest include green vegetables, whole grains, beans, lentils, and peas. In addition, they most often include fiber, which not only slows down digestion but also keeps you feeling fuller longer, and they don't spike your blood sugar levels.

In fact, these carbohydrates may be your best friends, because they provide phytochemicals (plant-based nutrients) that help fight inflammation. When inflammation occurs on the outside of your body, you know it. Your skin turns red, and there may be swelling and sometimes pain. This kind of inflammation occurs in response to a wound or insult of some kind, such as a cut or a sunburn. It is a sign that your body is trying to heal itself. When inflammation occurs internally, however, you probably won't know it, and it may occur because your body is responding to an internal threat you may not even know you have. If the cause of the problem is not addressed, the inflammation will persist and may begin to attack your organs or vital bodily functions. Chronic inflammation has been linked to an increased risk of heart attack and many other life-threatening diseases.

If you eat unhealthy foods over a long period of time, you create a buildup of unhealthy bacteria in your gut, and in response, your body activates an inflammatory response to try to destroy the bacteria. But if you keep eating more of those unhealthy foods, your body will continue to attack those bacteria and your gut will be chronically inflamed.

In addition to eating foods such as fish that are rich in omega-3 fatty acids, one of the simplest and most effective ways to reduce or eliminate internal inflammation is to increase your intake of colorful fruits and vegetables, which are rich in polyphenols, chemicals found in plant-based foods that fight inflammation.

Don't Stress About Your Food

We're all going to eat something we know isn't healthy at one time or another. So long as your diet isn't made up entirely, or even mainly, of unhealthy foods, I say eat it, enjoy it, and then forget about it. Stressing or feeling guilty about your "slip up" isn't going to change anything—except that it will increase the amount of the stress hormone cortisol in your system, which will probably make you want to eat even more bad stuff to soothe yourself.

Get Your Vitamins and Minerals from Foods

Vitamins are organic elements that can be negatively affected by cooking, processing, and exposure to light. Minerals are inorganic elements found in the soil, which means that they are not generally affected by food preparation. Both vitamins and minerals are essential nutrients because they act in concert with one another to perform hundreds of important functions in your body. They are called micronutrients because you require only small quantities to remain healthy. A lack of any one, however, could lead to serious health problems, such as scurvy (from a lack of vitamin C), rickets (from a lack of vitamin D), and even blindness (from a lack vitamin A), to name just a few. Minerals are also important for maintaining good health. For example, you need calcium for strong bones, iron to enrich your blood, and potassium to ensure heart health.

Vitamins and minerals interact with one another in extremely complex ways. Too much or too little of one could inhibit the maximum function of another. Too much sodium, for example, mainly from eating too many processed foods, could reduce your calcium levels, because calcium binds with sodium and is excreted when your body senses a sodium overload.[18]

Getting too much of any of these micronutrients generally results from taking too many supplements. If you follow the food plan I'll be giving you, you will be getting all the vitamins and minerals you need from the foods you eat, which is a lot healthier than taking supplements to make up for those you're not getting because you're not eating the most nutritious foods.

The Exception to the Vitamin and Mineral Rule

We need vitamin B_{12} to perform many essential functions, such as making red blood cells, but some people don't get enough while others can't absorb what they do get through diet. Because it is found only in animal products, strict vegetarians and vegans are often B_{12} deficient. And some older people, as well as those who take certain medications, are not able to absorb B_{12} no matter how many animal products they eat. So, in particular circumstances, some people do need to take supplements of this important micronutrient even if they are following a healthy diet.[19]

ReSYNC Lite—Easing into the Plan

Of course, I would like everyone to start the ReSYNC diet as soon as possible, but I've found that sometimes, after years of eating unhealthy foods, it's simply too radical a change for people to make all at once. When I see that one of my clients is finding it too difficult, I suggest a more gradual approach, which I call "ReSYNC Lite." Basically, it's taking one small step at a time, mainly to drastically reduce the amount of sugar in one's diet, so that the body is prepared to follow the ReSYNC diet. The bottom line is that I don't want anyone to fail, so I work with people to make sure they will succeed.

One of those clients was Sarah. She was a thirty-seven-year-old teacher, married, with a thirteen-year-old daughter. Sarah had been overweight her entire life. Now she had type 2 diabetes, and her family was following in her footsteps. Her husband was also overweight, and her daughter was prediabetic.

Sarah really wanted to get healthy and was trying her hardest to follow the ReSYNC diet, but after two weeks I realized it wasn't working for her. Making changes all at once was just too hard for her. So I told her we were going to change her plan. I explained that I would give her twenty-eight simple steps to ease into the diet. She could add one step a day for twenty-eight days, or, if she felt she could do more, she could add steps more quickly and be ready to move on even sooner. Sarah took the entire four weeks to implement all the steps, and at the end of that time she had lost only seven pounds. But she was feeling stronger, she no longer had sugar cravings, and she was ready to move on.

She started on the ReSYNC diet, but it still wasn't working as well as we both thought it should. Her husband and daughter were still eating the way they always had and were bringing sugary snacks into the house. With their agreement, I put them both on the ReSYNC Lite plan while Sarah was on the regular diet. Finally, the whole family was on their way to better health. Sarah lost twenty-two pounds in the next month, and after three more months she had lost a total of fifty-seven pounds.

Now Sarah is maintaining a healthy weight of 140 pounds. Her husband went from 230 to 185 pounds, and her daughter is also a healthy weight. Sarah's type 2 diabetes has completely resolved, and her daughter is no longer prediabetic. It is often the case—and always gratifying for me—that when one family member starts to get fit, the entire family benefits.

If you're afraid that plunging into the ReSYNC diet all at once is too much, follow these twenty-eight ReSYNC Lite steps:

1. **Set daily goals and reward yourself for meeting them.** To a sugar addict, nothing is tougher than getting through the day without a sugary treat. The longer you can hold out, the easier it will become, so try to find a reward that would be worth holding out for.

2. **Drink plenty of water.** Every time you feel hungry or have a sugar craving, drink a big glass of water and wait ten minutes. More often than not, your craving will pass. We sometimes mistake thirst for hunger, and you may be craving sugar because you're dehydrated. You should be drinking twelve to fourteen glasses of water every day.

3. **Walk around the block.** Research shows that physical activity can curb cravings for sweets. Exercise produces endorphins, which boost your mood and energy, and decreases stress, reducing the likelihood that you'll engage in stress-induced eating. Exercise also improves insulin sensitivity in skeletal muscle, lowering insulin levels in the bloodstream.

4. **Eat five times a day.** You should eat three small, healthy meals and two snacks throughout the day. Eating small meals containing lean protein, complex carbohydrates, and healthy fats can help stabilize your blood sugar, which will eliminate your cravings. If you need to skip a meal, skip dinner instead of breakfast. You need breakfast to give you energy to get you going in the morning.

5. **Avoid artificial sweeteners.** They are not a solution to avoiding or

decreasing sugar cravings. They may taste sweet, but they don't fool the brain into producing the pleasure chemicals sugar does, so they might actually increase your sugar craving instead of satisfying it.

6. **Stay away from sports drinks.** They have just as much, if not more, sugar than soda.

7. **Eat sweet vegetables.** If you include more sweet vegetables, such as sweet potatoes, carrots, beets, and bell peppers in your diet, you will naturally crave less sugar. Eat them cooked to release their maximum sweetness.

8. **Treat yourself to a healthy dessert.** A bowl of fruit with Greek yogurt makes an ideal dessert. The fruit is sweet and contains vitamins and minerals as well as fiber to help fill you up. Yogurt adds a creamy texture along with calcium for strong bones. Here are some great combinations:

   - Fresh pineapple, banana, orange, and melon mixed with honey and yogurt
   - Dried apricots, figs, and dates served with a dollop of Greek yogurt
   - Frozen berries, grapes, and banana blended with Greek yogurt to make a fruity frozen dessert

9. **Eat less.** Instead of giving up sugar "cold turkey," start slowly reducing the *volume* of sugar you eat each day. If you typically add two teaspoons of sugar to your coffee, try cutting back to just one (or even one and a half). If you usually drink five glasses of soda each day, try drinking only a half glass for each full glass you would normally drink.

10. **Indulge less often.** Once you feel more comfortable with a reduced volume of sugar, you can also start consuming it less often. Replace two or three glasses of soda with water. Have sugar in one cup of coffee but not in the others you drink later in the day. You may start out consuming sugar a

dozen times a day and gradually cut down to only once or twice a day—or even stop altogether.

11. **Switch to dark chocolate.** It contains less sugar than milk chocolate and is rich in antioxidants. Look for options that contain at least 75 percent cacao.

12. **Switch to whole-grain bread.** It's much less likely than refined white bread to spike your blood sugar and therefore your cravings.

13. **Eat nuts.** Highly nutritious and energy dense, nuts are the perfect food to ward off cravings. Some nuts, such as raw cashews and macadamia nuts, also taste sweet and creamy, giving the illusion of having a sweet treat. Numerous studies show that people who eat a small quantity of nuts in a day are slenderer than those who don't eat any nuts at all.

14. **Flavor with spices.**

    - Cinnamon can help curb your sweet tooth almost instantly. It has a natural sweet taste and has been shown to lower the glycemic index of other foods when eaten with them.

    - Cayenne does not taste sweet but has been proven to curb appetite and a sweet tooth. Because its flavor is so intense, the tongue is satisfied very quickly, and you won't crave sugar after eating it. I like to use cayenne along with lemon in my morning tea.

    - Ginger is a rock star spice that I hope you're already using. Ginger is strong and spicy, with sweet undertones that work well with other spices, such as cinnamon, nutmeg, and cardamom, which are naturally sweet tasting. It wakes you up and rejuvenates your whole body so you won't need to turn to sugar for that sense of alertness.

15. **Eat plenty of greens.** Nutrient-rich green drinks can increase energy levels and reduce sugar and processed food cravings. (See the Green Smoothie recipe.)

GREEN SMOOTHIE

Here's a recipe for a super-nourishing smoothie.

1 cup coconut water

1/2 cup loosely packed cilantro

1 cup loosely packed organic baby kale (or another baby green)

1 cup loosely packed organic spinach

1 cup cucumber, roughly chopped

1/2 cup pineapple cubes

1/2 green apple, cored and roughly chopped

Juice of 1 lemon or lime

1/4 avocado, peeled and roughly chopped

1 teaspoon flax seeds (optional)

1 teaspoon hemp seeds (optional)

Combine all ingredients in blender and process until smooth, about 60 seconds. Add flax seeds and hemp seeds, if using, and blend briefly again.

Makes one smoothie.

16. **Eat more protein.** Cravings for sugar are often caused by a dip in blood sugar levels, and eating protein regularly helps stabilize your blood sugar by increasing the length of time it takes to metabolize your food.

17. **Get more vitamins C and B complex.** Among other important duties, vitamin C helps convert tryptophan (from the food you eat) into serotonin. B-complex vitamins help you metabolize carbohydrates for the body to use as energy. Foods that are high in vitamin C include yellow and red bell peppers, kale, broccoli, and kiwis. Fish and shellfish, calves' liver, white meat chicken, and low-fat cheese are all good sources of B vitamins.

18. **Drink green tea.** It contains antioxidants that will help regulate blood sugar levels and increase your metabolism and burn fat.

19. **Eat aromatic foods.** Strong aromas (spicy, meaty, peppery, buttery, lemony, oniony) wake up the hypothalamus—the part of your brain that tells you it's time to stop munching.

20. **Enjoy fermented foods and drinks.** Probiotic-rich fermented foods and drinks, such as yogurt, tempeh, pickles, sauerkraut, and miso soup, to name a few, can effectively eliminate sugar cravings, sometimes in just four to five days.

21. **Look out for hidden sugars.** Ketchup, barbecue sauce, tomato sauce, baked beans, salad dressings, breads, and lunch meats are just a few of the items that can contain a large amount of added sugar.

22. **Cut down on red meat.** Red meat is high in a pro-inflammatory molecule called *arachidonic acid*. Eating a lot of meat tends to increase the oxidative-inflammatory cascade in your body. If left unchecked, this inflammatory condition can become chronic and cause abnormal glucose metabolism, ultimately leading to insulin resistance.

23. **Avoid processed foods.** Studies have shown that eating processed foods, which tend to be high in sugar, sodium, and fat, can be as addictive as heroin or morphine, leading to cravings, overeating, and obesity.

24. **Stay away from "low-fat" desserts.** They generally contain added sugar to compensate for the flavor that is lost with the reduction of fat.

25. **Eat a real meal.** If you are craving something sweet, check to see if you are just hungry. Eating a real, healthy meal can decrease sweet cravings triggered by low energy.

26. **Let your family help.** If you must have cookies in the house, ask your partner to stash them where you can't see them. Have your teenager put away the butter pecan ice cream so it's not the first thing you see when

you open the freezer. It doesn't help to come face-to-face with temptation when you're looking for the frozen lima beans.

27. **Avoid boredom.** It's one of the main craving triggers. When you're home, try knitting, reading, drawing, or playing video games or a board game with a family member. Engaging in activities that keep your hands busy is a good way to take your mind off food.

28. **Meditate or pray.** Daily prayer or meditation can reduce stress and minimize sugar cravings.

The Twenty-Eight-Day ReSYNC Diet Plan

My hope is that you'll be able to move into the ReSYNC diet plan right away, as my client Richard did. When I met him, Richard was fifty-eight years old, five feet eight inches tall, and weighed 250 pounds. He told me that he was very unhappy because he'd been fit all his life until he was in a serious car accident about a year before and had to stop working out. In his own mind, Richard still thought of himself as someone who was very fit, but he no longer had the mental acuity to do what he knew he needed to do to be fit. As a chemical engineer and an executive vice president of his company, he was used to managing multimillion-dollar projects, being in charge, commanding respect, and motivating people on his team.

Now, he told me, he was still acting the part of the "take charge" leader, but he no longer felt that way inside. Instead, he felt that he was acting the part but not really feeling it. He didn't feel as mentally sharp as he had been, and he hated the feeling that he was losing his edge.

The fact that he could no longer bench-press or lift the amount of weight he used to was a wake-up call for him. For the first couple of weeks he was working with me, he actually felt depressed, because until then he hadn't realized how out of shape he really was. My job was to pick up his spirits and remind him that he was just out of practice and needed to get back on the proverbial horse.

Richard was already extremely determined and highly motivated to succeed. In fact, he was one of my few clients who did absolutely everything I asked of him. Within the first month, he was well on his way to getting back to his pre-accident weight. Within nine months he was down to 163 pounds, which was significantly less than he had weighed before the accident. He felt strong and in charge again, and he told me that until he had allowed himself to get out of shape and then regained his fitness, he hadn't appreciated how important fitness was not only for his physical health but also for his business and social interactions.

Richard was motivated to regain his competitive edge, but other people are motivated by many other things. Do you want to look younger? Do you want to have more energy to play with your children or grandchildren? Do you want to have a better social life? Do you want to wow your classmates at your next high school reunion? Whatever it is—and no one reason is better than any other—you have to find what's going to motivate you.

Start Today

The ReSYNC diet plan is an easy-to-follow guide for eating well while eliminating foods that may be sapping your energy and preventing you from being as lean and healthy as I know you can be. As you will see, the plan is divided into four weekly segments, and each segment contains five different food lists. The first list (Daily Requirements) specifies the foods and beverages you need to have every single day. That is followed by a selection of snacks from which you will choose one in the morning and one in the afternoon.

The last three lists indicate the proteins, carbs, and fats you can mix and match to create your own menus for breakfast, lunch, and dinner. You can prepare them any way you like, so long as you use only the ingredients listed and stick to the specified portion sizes.

The first week is the most restrictive because it is designed to reenergize your digestive system, clear your gut of any toxins that may have been accumulating over time, and jump-start your weight loss.

You will see that more foods, and in some cases increased portion sizes, are added each week. By the end of week four, you'll be ready to move on to the ReSYNC for Life program described in chapter 7.

Following the food lists, you will find suggestions for three meals and two snacks that are appropriate for each of the four weeks of the diet. Remember, these are just suggestions. You don't have to use my menus or cook the foods exactly as I describe. So long as you stick to these simple rules, you'll be leaner and feeling fitter with each passing week. And remember these important tips:

- Don't skip breakfast.
- When you feel hungry, drink two glasses of water and wait ten to twenty minutes. If you are still hungry, have a snack.
- Your last meal of the day should be at least ninety minutes before you go to sleep.
- Drink your water!
- Chew slowly, focus on the texture and taste, and take your time with your food.

Week One: Daily Requirements

Water: 6 or more 10-ounce glasses of water a day including 10 ounces of water with lemon or lime 20 minutes before each meal and 30 minutes after each meal. In addition, drink a 10-ounce glass of water with lemon or lime after each cup of coffee you drink.

Green tea: 1 to 3 cups daily (drink 10 ounces of water after each cup)

1 grapefruit for breakfast

Recommended: Hot pepper or cayenne pepper in some form, in any dish

Week One: Snack Options

Choose one morning and one afternoon snack.

1 cucumber with lemon juice

3 ribs celery

1 green apple

1 cup berries

1 cup nonfat Greek yogurt

Week One: Protein Options

Wild white fish, such as cod, tilapia, halibut, catfish, bass, flounder, haddock, mahi-mahi, monkfish, perch, shark, skate, snapper, swordfish, trout (6 ounces)

Skinless chicken breast (6 ounces)

Eggs (2 whole or 4 whites)

Tofu and/or tempeh, only if vegetarian or vegan (3/4 cup)

Week One: Carb Options

Unlimited serving size, unless otherwise indicated.

Any leafy greens, such as kale, spinach, arugula, collards, and chard

Any lettuces

All green vegetables, such as zucchini, broccoli, bok choy, green beans, peas, Brussels sprouts, cucumber, celery, cabbage, fennel, and kohlrabi

Berries, such as strawberries, blueberries, raspberries, blackberries, and acai berries

Tomatoes, yellow squash, bell pepper (1 cup)

Green apples

Mestemacher Fitness Bread (available at markets such as Whole Foods and online) or other dense, chewy, dark, high-fiber bread (½ slice per day, preferably with breakfast or lunch)

Raw oats (½ cup)

Week One: Fat Options

Almond or coconut milk (1 cup per day)

Oils, such as coconut oil, avocado oil, walnut oil, extra-virgin olive oil, and flaxseed oil (1 tablespoon per serving)

Flax seeds or pumpkin seeds (1 tablespoon)

Almonds or walnuts (8 to 12 nuts)

Week Two: Daily Requirements

Water: 6 or more 10-ounce glasses of water a day including 10 ounces of water with lemon or lime 20 minutes before each meal and 30 minutes after each meal. In addition, drink a 10-ounce glass of water with lemon or lime after each cup of coffee you drink.

Green tea: 1 to 3 cups daily (drink 10 ounces of water after each cup)

1 grapefruit

Recommended: Hot pepper or cayenne pepper in some form, in any dish

Week Two: Snack Options

Choose one morning and one afternoon snack. In addition to the snacks listed for week one, you can enjoy the following:

Edamame ($\frac{1}{2}$ cup)

8 to 12 almonds, walnuts, pine nuts, or Brazil nuts

$\frac{1}{2}$ green apple with 1 tablespoon almond butter

$\frac{1}{2}$ banana

1 cup melon

2 ribs celery with 1 tablespoon hummus

Week Two: Protein Options

Four ounces per serving unless otherwise indicated. In addition to the proteins listed for week one, you can have the following:

Skinless white-meat turkey

Squid

Tuna

Salmon

Clams (4 ounces of meat)

Shrimp

Scallops

Sardines in water

Navy beans, black beans, pinto beans, lentils, split peas, mungo beans
($\frac{1}{2}$ cup)

Cottage cheese (1 cup)

Week Two: Carb Options

Unlimited serving size, unless otherwise indicated. In addition to the carb options listed for week one, you can enjoy the following:

Eggplant, mushrooms, beets, turnips, radishes, carrots, Swiss chard,
cauliflower, okra, artichoke (1 cup)

Citrus fruits, such as oranges, clementines, and grapefruit (1 per day)

Orchard fruits, especially apples and pears (1 per day)

Melons, such as watermelon, cantaloupe, and honeydew melon (1 cup)

Banana (½, as breakfast)

Quinoa, couscous, buckwheat, bulgur, and rye (½ cup cooked)

Week Two: Fat Options

In addition to the fat options listed for week one, you can enjoy:

Avocado (½)

Hummus (¼ cup)

Almond butter (1 tablespoon)

Pine nuts, Brazil nuts (8 to 12 nuts)

Seeds, such as sunflower seeds, pumpkin seeds, chia seeds, poppy seeds, sesame seeds (1 tablespoon)

Week Three: Daily Requirements

Water: 8 or more 10-ounce glasses of water a day including 10 ounces of water with lemon or lime 20 minutes before each meal and 30 minutes after each meal. In addition, drink a 10-ounce glass of water with lemon or lime after each cup of coffee you drink.

Green tea: 1 to 3 cups daily (drink 10 ounces of water after each cup)

1 grapefruit

Recommended: Hot pepper or cayenne pepper in some form, in any dish

Week Three: Snack Options

Choose one morning and one afternoon snack. In addition to the snack options listed for weeks one and two, you can enjoy the following:

¹/₂ green apple or pear with 1 tablespoon natural peanut butter

4 green or black olives

¹/₃ ounce 75 percent cacao dark chocolate

1 cup cherries

1 cup grapes

1 carrot drizzled with lemon juice

Week Three: Protein Options

Four ounces per serving unless otherwise indicated. In addition to the proteins listed for weeks one and two, you can enjoy the following:

Calves' liver or beef liver

Bison or buffalo meat

Venison

Week Three: Carb Options

Unlimited serving size, unless otherwise indicated. In addition to the carb options listed for weeks one and two, you can enjoy the following:

Sweet potatoes, yams, butternut squash, acorn squash, spaghetti squash, or pumpkin (¹/₂ cup)

Pineapple, papaya, or mango (¹/₂ cup)

Peaches, nectarines, or kiwi (1 per day)

Apricots (3 per day)

Bread: 100 percent whole-wheat or 100 percent whole-grain (1 slice). Note that the sodium content needs to be less than 180mg per slice.

Week Three: Fat Options

In addition to the fat options listed for weeks one and two, you can enjoy the following:

Dark chocolate, minimum 75 percent cacao (1/3 to 1/2 ounce)

Sunflower oil, borage oil (1 to 2 tablespoons)

Natural peanut butter (1 tablespoon)

Organic peanuts (1/2 to 1 ounce)

Olives (4)

Cheese: parmesan (1 tablespoon, grated) or mozzarella, goat cheese, Camembert cheese (1 ounce)

Week Four: Daily Requirements

Water: 10 or more 10-ounce glasses of water a day including 10 ounces of water with lemon or lime 20 minutes before each meal and 30 minutes after each meal. In addition, drink a 10-ounce glass of water with lemon or lime after each cup of coffee you drink.

Green tea: 1 to 3 cups daily (drink 10 ounces of water after each cup)

1 grapefruit

Recommended: Hot pepper or cayenne pepper in some form, in any dish

Week Four: Snack Options

Choose one morning and one afternoon snack. In addition to the snack options listed for weeks one, two, and three, you can enjoy the following:

Dried fruit (2 to 3 pieces or a small handful of raisins)

1/2 apple with 1 ounce mozzarella, Camembert, or goat cheese

Week Four: Protein Options

Four ounces per serving unless otherwise indicated. In addition to the protein options for weeks one, two, and three, you can enjoy the following:

Beef, such as eye of round, sirloin tip side steak, top sirloin, bottom
round, filet mignon, skirt steak

Pork, such as pork tenderloin, rib chops, sirloin roast, top-loin chops

Week Four: Carb Options

Unlimited serving size, unless otherwise indicated. In addition to the carb
options for weeks one, two, and three, you can enjoy the following:

Brown rice, wild rice, black rice ($\frac{1}{2}$ cup cooked)

Buckwheat pasta, spelt pasta, quinoa pasta, multigrain pasta ($\frac{1}{2}$ cup,
cooked)

Dried fruit (2 to 3 pieces or a small handful of raisins)

Banana (1 a day, only at breakfast)

Week Four: Fat Options

Enjoy any of the fats listed for weeks one, two, and three.

Free Additions for All Weeks

Use any of the following foods and condiments with your meals:

Mustard (all types)

Vinegar (all types, but apple cider vinegar is recommended)

Onions and garlic

Sea salt

Any type of pepper

Hot sauce (such as Tabasco or sriracha)

Salsa, red or green ($\frac{1}{4}$ cup)

Reduced-sodium broth or stock (chicken, turkey, or veggie)

Lemon and lime

Herbs for seasoning

Stevia

Coffee (black, or add almond milk and/or stevia). Remember to always follow each cup of coffee with 15 ounces of water with lemon or lime, and alternate coffee with green tea.

Dressing Suggestions

These low-fat dressings may be used in salads or as a garnish for your protein and carb selections.

BASIL PESTO

1 cup fresh basil

2 tablespoons pine nuts

1/2 avocado

1 garlic clove

Juice of 1/2 lemon

3 tablespoons water

Combine all ingredients in food processor and pulse for 20 seconds.

Makes about 3/4 cup.

CILANTRO YOGURT DRESSING

1 cup chopped cilantro

$1/2$ cup Greek yogurt

1 garlic clove, pressed

2 teaspoons olive oil

Juice of 1 lemon

Salt and pepper to taste

Combine all ingredients and mix well.

Makes about $3/4$ cup.

DIJON MUSTARD DRESSING

1 teaspoon olive oil

$1/2$ teaspoon Dijon mustard

1 teaspoon organic apple cider vinegar

Salt and pepper to taste

Combine all ingredients and mix well.

Makes about $2 1/2$ teaspoons.

Week One Menu Suggestions
Breakfast

In addition to your citrus water, coffee or tea, and grapefruit, choose one of these three options:

1. Berry Yogurt. Mix Greek yogurt with berries and flax seeds
2. Veggie Eggs. Two eggs, $1/2$ slice of Mestemacher Fitness Bread, and a side of tomatoes and cucumbers

3. Breakfast Smoothie. Blend 1 cup Greek yogurt, 1 cup frozen berries, 1 teaspoon flaxseed, and 1 cup ice.

Morning Snack

Choose one from the list of week one snack options.

Lunch

In addition to citrus water and green tea (if drinking it with lunch), choose one of these three options:

1. Chicken and Veggies. 6 ounces poached boneless, skinless chicken breast, chopped or shredded, combined with 1 cup cherry tomatoes, 1 teaspoon chopped sun-dried tomato, and ½ cup raw or blanched chopped asparagus spears. Season with salt, pepper, and fresh basil.
2. Chicken and Vegetable Soup. Soup made with reduced-sodium chicken broth, chopped cooked chicken breast, and chopped vegetables from the week one carb options. Serve with leafy greens of your choice sautéed in 1 tablespoon olive oil and seasoned with cayenne pepper.
3. Snapper and Veggies. 4 ounces grilled snapper fillet served with grilled mixed vegetables from the week one carb options.

Afternoon Snack

Choose one from the list of week one snack options.

Dinner

In addition to citrus water, choose one of these three options:

1. Lemon Chicken. 6 ounces grilled boneless, skinless chicken breast served with grilled vegetables from the week one carb options, sprinkled with finely grated lemon zest and chopped fresh thyme.

2. Grilled Halibut. 4 ounces grilled halibut, seasoned with cayenne pepper and served with steamed broccoli and a side salad dressed with 1 tablespoon of olive oil and balsamic vinegar.

3. Grilled Fish Tacos. 4 ounces of fish of your choice, diced tomato, green peppers, and onions, seasoned with cayenne pepper and wrapped in lettuce leaves.

Week Two Menu Suggestions

Breakfast

In addition to your citrus water, coffee or tea, and grapefruit, choose one of these three options:

1. Poached Eggs. Two poached eggs with grilled or steamed asparagus.

2. Egg White Omelet. Combine 4 egg whites, chopped bell pepper, celery, onions, and tomatoes, and serve with ½ slice Mestamacher Fitness Bread.

3. Veggie Quiche Cup. Chop a mix of your favorite veggies and place in muffin cup, filling it halfway. In bowl, whisk 2 eggs with salt and pepper (add herbs of your choice if desired), and pour over veggies, filling muffin cup to within ¼ inch of top. Bake for 20 to 25 minutes at 350 degrees. Scoop onto plate and enjoy.

Morning Snack

Choose one from the lists of weeks one or two snack options.

Lunch

In addition to citrus water and green tea (if drinking it with lunch), choose one of these three options:

1. Tomato Soup Smoothie. In blender, combine 2 large, ripe, peeled

tomatoes, 1 cup plain Greek yogurt, and a pinch of fresh basil. Blend until smooth and season with salt and pepper.

2. Chicken and Cabbage. Combine 2 cups shredded cabbage with 1 cup shredded carrots. Toss with 1 teaspoon olive oil, lemon juice to taste, and 2 tablespoons chopped fresh dill. Top with 4 ounces grilled skinless, boneless chicken breast.

3. Roasted Cauliflower. Toss florets from ¼-head cauliflower with 1 teaspoon olive oil, 1 chopped garlic clove, salt, and pepper, and roast for 20 minutes at 450 degrees. Serve with 4 ounces grilled shrimp and 2 teaspoons Cilantro Yogurt Dressing (page 88).

Afternoon Snack

Choose one from the lists of weeks one or two snack options.

Dinner

In addition to citrus water, choose one of these three options:

1. Tuna with Green Beans and Almonds. Heat 1 tablespoon olive oil in skillet over medium-high heat. Season 4-ounce tuna fillet with salt and pepper, and roll it in sesame seeds. Add fish to pan and cook for 2 to 3 minutes on each side. In second pan, heat 1 tablespoon olive oil. When hot, add 1 chopped garlic clove, a large handful of green beans, and ¼ cup sliced almonds. Season with sea salt and cook, stirring occasionally, until beans are crisp-tender, for 3 to 5 minutes. Serve beans with tuna.

2. Grilled Chicken Breast with Brussels Sprouts. Heat 1 tablespoon olive oil in skillet over medium-high heat. Add chopped Brussels sprouts and cook, stirring, until softened. Add 1 teaspoon chopped walnuts

and season with Dijon Mustard Dressing (page 89). Serve with 4 ounces grilled skinless, boneless chicken breast.

3. Grilled Portobello Mushrooms with Tomatoes and Eggplant. Season two Portobello mushrooms with sea salt and olive oil and grill over medium-high heat for 10 minutes. Heat 1 tablespoon olive oil in skillet. When hot, add 1 cup chopped onion and 2 chopped garlic cloves. Cook, stirring until onion is golden brown. Add 2 cups chopped tomato and 1 cup chopped eggplant, and cook, stirring, for another 5 to 10 minutes. To serve, top mushrooms with onion and tomato mixture.

Week Three Menu Suggestions
Breakfast

In addition to your citrus water, coffee or tea, and grapefruit, choose one of these three options:

1. Overnight Oatmeal. In container with tight-fitting lid, combine ½ cup raw oats, ½ cup nonfat milk or almond milk, and 1 teaspoon honey. Shake to mix well and refrigerate overnight. In the morning, when ready to eat, add 1 cup fresh berries and 1 teaspoon chopped mixed nuts.

2. Banana-Chia Smoothie. In a container with a tight-fitting lid, combine ¼ cup chia seeds with ½ cup almond milk and ½ cup coconut milk. Shake to mix well and refrigerate overnight. In the morning, when ready to eat, add ½ chopped banana and 1 teaspoon sliced almonds.

3. Fruit and Cottage Cheese. Combine 1 cup cottage cheese with ⅓ cup chopped plums and 1 tablespoon chopped walnuts.

Morning Snack

Choose one from the lists of weeks one, two, and three snack options.

Lunch

In addition to citrus water and green tea (if drinking it with lunch), choose one of these three options:

1. Turkey and Lettuce Bowl. In skillet over medium heat, sauté ½ chopped yellow onion in 1 teaspoon olive oil until soft but not brown. Add 3 ounces ground lean turkey and cook, stirring, until meat is no longer pink. Season with salt and cayenne pepper, and serve in bowl over shredded lettuce, chopped tomatoes, and peppers.

2. Fish and Sweet Potatoes. 4 ounces grilled cod fillet served with ½ cup sweet potato purée.

3. Broccoli and Kale Soup. Heat 1 tablespoon olive oil in large skillet over medium-high heat. Add 1 chopped garlic clove, 1 teaspoon chopped fresh ginger, ½ teaspoon turmeric, salt and pepper to taste, and cook, stirring, 1 to 2 minutes. Add 2 cups low-sodium vegetable broth and cook 5 minutes more. Add 1 cup broccoli florets and 2 to 3 cups chopped kale, and cook until broccoli is crisp-tender, 4 to 5 more minutes. Serve in soup bowl, and season with chopped cilantro and lime juice.

Afternoon Snack

Choose one from the lists of weeks one, two, and three snack options.

Dinner

In addition to citrus water and green tea (if drinking it with dinner), choose one of these three options:

1. Quinoa and Scallops. Combine ½ cup cooked quinoa with ¼ cup chickpeas, ½ cucumber, cut into cubes, and ¼ head cabbage, shredded.

Season with lemon juice and dill (or another herb of your choice), and serve with 3½ ounces grilled scallops.

2. Spaghetti Squash with Tomatoes. Preheat oven to 400 degrees. Cut a spaghetti squash in half and remove seeds. Roast squash for 25 to 40 minutes, until flesh is tender and skin is easily pierced with fork. Use fork to scrape out squash so that it forms spaghetti-like strands. Heat 1 tablespoon olive oil in skillet over medium-high heat. When hot, add ½ cup cherry tomato halves and cook, stirring, for 3 to 5 minutes. Season with salt and pepper. Add 1 chopped garlic clove and spaghetti squash. Cook, stirring, for 2 minutes longer. Remove from heat and stir in ½ cup cubed fresh mozzarella cheese. Garnish with snipped fresh basil. Serve with 4 ounces grilled shrimp.

3. Chicken and Broccoli. 4 ounces grilled skinless, boneless chicken breast served with grilled or steamed broccoli florets and carrots seasoned with salt and pepper.

Week Four Menu Suggestions

Breakfast

In addition to your citrus water, coffee or tea, and grapefruit, choose one of these three options:

1. Rice and Egg Bowl. Place ½ cup cooked brown rice in bowl. Top with two poached eggs and ½ avocado, sliced. Season with salt, pepper, and minced green onions.

2. Banana-Berry Smoothie. In blender, combine 1 banana, 1 cup almond milk, 1 cup fresh or frozen berries, 1 tablespoon flaxseeds, and 1 cup ice. Blend for 60 seconds.

3. Egg and Vegetable Stovetop Frittata. Steam 1 cup chopped mixed vegetables (whatever is fresh and available) for 2 to 3 minutes. In bowl,

beat 2 eggs with salt and pepper. Heat nonstick skillet over medium heat. Add vegetables and pour eggs on top. Cover skillet and cook for another 2 minutes (until eggs are done to your taste). Serve with a slice of whole-grain bread.

Morning Snack

Choose one from the lists of weeks one, two, three, or four snack options.

Lunch

In addition to citrus water and green tea (if drinking it with lunch), choose one of these three options:

1. Steak and Cukes. 4 ounces grilled top sirloin or sirloin tip steak served with a side of thinly sliced cucumber, sprinkled with 1 tablespoon sesame seeds and dressed with apple cider vinegar, olive oil, salt, and pepper.
2. Quinoa Fruit Bowl. Combine ½ cup cooked red quinoa with 1 sliced pear, 2½ ounces fresh baby spinach, and ¼ cup dried cranberries. Season with lemon juice, salt, and pepper. Serve with 4 ounces grilled chicken.
3. Pasta and Tomatoes. Heat 1 tablespoon olive oil in skillet over medium heat. Add ½ cup cooked buckwheat pasta, 5 or 6 cherry tomatoes, and 1 teaspoon chopped olives. Cook, stirring, for about 3 minutes. Season with salt, pepper, and fresh basil. Serve with 4 ounces grilled shrimp.

Afternoon Snack

Choose one from the lists of weeks one, two, three, or four snack options.

Dinner

In addition to citrus water and green tea (if drinking it with dinner), choose one of these three options:

1. Scallops and Vegetables. Heat 1 tablespoon olive oil in skillet over medium-high heat. Add ½ cup chopped onion and cook, stirring, until golden brown. Add 1 cup diced sweet potato and cook 15 to 20 minutes. Add 4 ounces scallops and cook 4 to 5 minutes, turning to brown both sides. When done, remove from the heat and add 2 cups chopped kale. Stir to combine.

2. Burger Salad. 4-ounce burger made with ground top or bottom round steak, served over a mixed green salad, dressed with olive oil and apple cider vinegar.

3. Pesto Pork Chop. Marinate a 4-ounce rib or loin pork chop in Basil Pesto (page 88) for 30 minutes; then grill over medium-high heat for 5 to 6 minutes on each side. Serve with grilled vegetables of your choice.

CHAPTER 4

ReSYNC Your Brain: Twenty-Eight Days to Smart

Since ancient times man has been fascinated by the workings of the human brain. The first description of brain anatomy and the effects of brain injury on other parts of the body appears in the Edwin Smith Surgical Papyrus, dating to about 1600 BC.[1] Alcmaeon, an early Greek medical writer and philosopher-scientist, was the first to write that the brain is the seat of understanding.[2]

I think you'll be amazed by how much we've learned since those early times about how the brain works, and by how much you can do, simply by changing your diet and ramping up your exercise regimen, to increase your own brainpower and keep yourself mentally fit for life.

Certainly there are differences in mental acuity between one person and the next. We are born with a certain level of biological intelligence. And some people are "smarter" in one area or another. But within those inborn parameters, your brain remains malleable throughout your life. According to Kevin McGrew, educational psychologist and director of the Institute for Applied Psychometrics, "It is possible to fine-tune your neural efficiency, or mental horsepower. Your cognitive functions can be made to work more efficiently and in a more synchronized manner."[3]

The movie *Limitless* is a sci-fi thriller in which a struggling writer is given an experimental "smart pill" called NZT-48, which, for a short period of time, gives him total recall and the ability to correlate all that he knows into useful information. Would you take that pill if it were offered to you?

Sure, that's science fiction—at least for now—although there are a handful of people we know about, such as the actress Marilu Henner, who can recall at will every day of their lives (a condition called *hyperthymesia*, or highly superior autobiographical memory). However, given the technology we already have to look inside the working brain, as well as the limitless fascination we have with how the biological supercomputers inside our heads actually work, I think that someday, sooner or later, we will all be able to tap into a level of brainpower that now seems out of reach.

Until that day, the ReSYNC Method is designed to maximize the functioning of our brains. Working with clients from every walk of life, including corporate executives, religious leaders, politicians, media personalities, and thousands of members of the general public, I have found that becoming more physically fit helps people develop more mental clarity and creativity and cope better with the stresses of daily life.

When we are stressed, our brain is focused on how to escape from the situation we are in, and as a result, we are not able to think about anything else. Reduction in our stress reaction therefore increases our ability to think more clearly about what we need to accomplish at work or in any other part of our lives.

I particularly remember David, an architect who came to me at his wife's insistence. David told me that his wife was very outgoing and took great pleasure in socializing with friends, but he was becoming extremely introverted. Over time, he'd been gaining weight almost without realizing it. And now, he said, he was slowing down, not only physically but mentally as well. He'd always been extremely focused on his work, but now it was taking him longer to solve problems he'd always been able to solve very quickly. In the past, he could always envision a project all the way to its conclusion, almost from the moment it was presented to him. Now, finding those solutions was taking a lot out of him. He felt that he was losing his mental acuity, and that made him feel like less of a man. The last thing he wanted to do after a long and exhausting day was go out and socialize. He hated parties because he could never remember anyone's name and he didn't have the mental energy to make small talk.

At the time, David, who is five feet eleven inches tall, weighed 235 pounds, and he wasn't doing any kind of exercise at all. Once I got him on the ReSYNC

Brain Bites ———————————————————————

Did you know?

- The adult human brain weighs about three pounds (1,300–1,400g), which is approximately 2 percent of total body weight.[4]
- More than one hundred thousand chemical reactions occur in the human brain every second.[5]
- In a lifetime your long-term memory can hold up to 1 quadrillion separate bits of information.[6]
- The brain of the Russian novelist Ivan Turgenev weighed 4.45 pounds (2,021 grams), about 70 percent more than average.[7]

program, he followed my instructions exactly—he was, after all, an architect and used to working with blueprints. He lost seventeen pounds in the first month, and three months later, he was down to 170 pounds. Within the first two weeks, he told me, he was already feeling stronger, and that gave his self-esteem a tremendous boost. Most important for both him and his wife, his brain fog lifted, and he was thinking clearly and creatively again, which meant that he was also less stressed, and even after a full day at work, he had the mental and physical energy to get up and go out.

Being Geniuses Together

Albert Einstein was widely quoted as saying that he went to his office at Princeton University's Institute for Advanced Study every day "just to have the privilege of walking home with Kurt Gödel."[8] When Einstein arrived at the institute, he was already fifty-four and his greatest discoveries were behind him. He had nothing to prove to anyone, and may have found some of his colleagues less than intellectually stimulating. But when Gödel, who has been called the greatest logician since Aristotle, arrived about a decade later, he and Einstein each found someone he considered an intellectual peer with whom he could talk seriously about the most complex scientific issues. Gödel was only in his thirties when Einstein was in his midsixties, but mentally, they were equals.

There is really no evidence to indicate that either Einstein or Gödel was walking because he thought it was "good for him." And there is nothing to show that they were walking "briskly," as most doctors and fitness experts would urge their clients to do. But as I've said, whatever physical exercise you can do will be for the good, and walking regularly, as these friends did twice a day every day (going to and from their respective offices) is a kind of exercise virtually anyone can do. In fact, I've found that when someone who comes to me is seriously overweight or sedentary, walking is about all he or she can do, and sometimes even that much exercise is difficult. But it's a start, and I've learned over time that it's important to start at whatever level my client can manage.

The Road to Getting Smarter: Take Your Brain for a Walk

Another great thinker, Friedrich Nietzsche, said, "All truly great thoughts are conceived by walking."[9] That may be a bit of an exaggeration, but many people say that walking helps them think more clearly, and there is significant scientific evidence to show that walking increases creative thought. A study by Marily Oppezzo and Daniel L. Schwartz at Stanford University indicates that in four different controlled scenarios, test subjects performed better on Guilford's Alternative Uses test for creative thinking when they were walking than they did while sitting.[10] And, in at least one of those scenarios, when the study participants were seated after walking, the effects of walking on the brain were still observable. The researchers concluded, "Walking opens up the free flow of ideas, and it is a simple and robust solution to the goals of increasing creativity and increasing physical activity."[11]

Use It, Don't Lose It

So walking stimulates the brain. However, it was not just the walking but undoubtedly also the ongoing use of their brain power that contributed to Einstein's and Gödel's extraordinary mind fitness. To keep your brain working at peak performance, you need to exercise it regularly.

A study by Sherry L. Willis, published in the *Journal of the American Medical Association (JAMA)*, showed that this "cognitive training improves cognitive function in well-functioning older adults and that this improvement lasts up to 5 years from the beginning of the intervention."[12] According to Richard J. Hodes, director of the National Institute on Aging, "The study addresses a very important hypothesis—that interventions can be designed to maintain cognitive function."[13]

Joe Verghese and colleagues at the Albert Einstein College of Medicine in Bronx, New York, studied the activities of 469 senior citizens and found that those who engaged in what might be considered time-wasting activities that challenge the mind, such as playing board games, solving crossword puzzles, or reading, were really not wasting time at all, because engaging in those sorts of activities was associated with a lower risk of developing dementia.[14]

Einstein's Brain

Einstein's brain weighed 1,230 grams or 2.71 pounds—less than the average adult brain, which weighs about 1,400 grams or 3.08 pounds. However, the density of neurons—cells that carry messages between the brain and other parts of the body—was greater.[15]

Friendship Boosts the Brain

In addition to exercising their bodies and their brains, Gödel and Einstein were reaping the rewards of social interaction. According to several studies, people with more social ties have been found to live longer, have better health, and be less depressed.[16]

If walking with Gödel was the sole reason Einstein bothered going to his office, undoubtedly that alone had a positive effect on his continued mental alertness. But if Jim Holt, author of the *New Yorker* magazine article "Time Bandits" is correct, Einstein did as much for Gödel, whom Holt describes as "solemn, solitary, and pessimistic."[17]

Friendships and social connections are important, but it's also important to choose your friends wisely. Surround yourself with people who believe in you, support you, and will help you get to the next level in your life. As for Gödel and Einstein, how fortunate for them that they found each other!

Walking Is Great, but More Is Better

Walking is definitely good exercise, but the more aerobic activity we incorporate into our lives, the better off we'll be, both mentally and physically. A study by Kirk I. Erickson of the University of Pittsburgh, published in the *Proceedings of the National Academy of Sciences*, found that regular aerobic exercise (the kind that really gets your heart pumping) can actually increase the size of the hippocampus, which is the area of the brain that is responsible for transferring information we receive into memory.[18]

Other experts support that claim too. Scott McGinnis, a neurologist at Boston's Brigham and Women's Hospital, confirms that "engaging in a program of regular exercise of moderate intensity over six months or a year is associated with an increase in the volume of selected brain regions."[19]

In addition, at least one study has shown that older adults (aged sixty to seventy-nine) who participated in aerobic training showed significant increases in brain volume after six months as compared to those who did only stretching and toning exercises. Stanley J. Colcombe at the University of Illinois and his fellow researchers concluded that "cardiovascular fitness is associated with the sparing of brain tissue in aging humans."[20]

And finally, in an observational study of 876 people who were enrolled in the Northern Manhattan Study (a research study of stroke and stroke risk factors in the Northern Manhattan community), Joshua Z. Willey and his fellow researchers found that among those who showed no signs of memory or thinking problems at the start of the study, those who reported low activity levels showed a greater decline over five years on tests that measured how fast they could perform simple tasks and how many words they could remember from a list, than those who reported high levels of activity. The difference was equal to that of ten years of aging.[21]

Furthermore, as we mentioned in chapter 1, regular exercise has been shown to reduce negative reactions to stress, probably through a series of chemical reactions in the body. Several studies support this finding, including one done by researchers at Princeton University and reported in the *Journal of Neuroscience*.[22]

Many of my own clients have also told me that until they began working out with the ReSYNC Method, they had trouble quieting their minds to fall asleep, and that they now sleep better and therefore wake up more focused and energized the next day. Several studies, including one by Helen S. Driver and Sheila R. Taylor, published in the *Sleep Medicine Reviews*,[23] have affirmed the connection between regular exercise and more deep sleep, but even without those studies, I can tell you that I know firsthand that it is true—and not because the people are more tired. As I saw with my client David and hundreds of others, exercise clears the mind, and once your mind is clear, you are able to stop worrying, relax, and get the sleep you need.

Learning from the Ancients

The phrase *mens sana in corpore sano*, or "a sound mind in a sound body," has been ascribed to the Roman poet Juvenal, who wrote in the late first and early second century AD. Whether or not the source is accurate (some have argued that the phrase was coined much earlier by the ancient philosopher Thales of Miletus[24]), the point is that the ancients understood that no one could really have a healthy mind without a healthy body, and vice versa.

Of course, health (both mental and physical) depends as much on proper nutrition as it does on regular exercise. Hippocrates, the ancient Greek physician who lived from about 460 to about 375 BC, is often quoted as having said, "If we could give every individual the right amount of nourishment and exercise, not too little and not too much, we would have found the safest way to health."

Food for Thought—Eat Your Way to Smarter

So how does that important fact relate to our friends Gödel and Einstein? As Holt points out in "Time Bandits," "Einstein freely indulged his appetite for heavy German cooking," while Gödel, who was obsessively concerned about his health, ironically followed a diet consisting of "butter, baby food, and laxatives."[25] So it's safe to say that neither of these great thinkers was applying his formidable intelligence to the proper nourishing of his brain.

Many studies have shown that what we eat affects the health of our minds. For example, a study by Martha Clare Morris and researchers at the Rush Institute for Healthy Aging of 815 people aged sixty-five and older found that both saturated fat and trans fat (the latter comes from a plant source and is transformed through a chemical process) were "positively associated with risk of Alzheimer's disease, whereas intakes of omega-6 polyunsaturated fat and monounsaturated fat were inversely associated. Persons in the upper fifth of saturated-fat intake had 2.2 times the risk of incident Alzheimer's disease compared with persons in the lowest fifth." The researchers concluded that "high intake of unsaturated, unhydrogenated fats may be protective against Alzheimer's disease, whereas intake of saturated or trans-unsaturated (hydrogenated) fats may increase risk."[26]

Ditch the Artificial Ingredients and Get Smarter

A study of one million students in New York City showed an improvement of about 14 percent on IQ tests after artificial flavors, preservatives, and dyes were removed from their lunch menu.[27]

We've all heard about the health benefits of following a Mediterranean diet, which is generally characterized as being rich in fruits, vegetables, nuts and grains, lean meats and fish, and by cooking with olive oil rather than butter. But now it appears that in addition to being heart healthy, this type of diet also protects the brain as we age. A cross-sectional study of 674 men eighty years or older that was conducted by Yian Gu and colleagues of the Taub Institute for Research in Alzheimer's Disease and the Aging Brain found that following a Mediterranean diet "was associated with less brain atrophy, with an effect similar to five years of aging. Higher fish and lower meat intake might be the two key food elements that contribute to the benefits" of this diet on brain structure.[28]

Stephanie Watson, executive editor of the *Harvard Women's Health Watch*, looked at a study done by researchers at the National Institute on Aging that also showed an association between eating a diet consisting of healthy nutrients (such as the Mediterranean diet) and better attention and memory skills. Perhaps more surprisingly, however, caffeine consumption was also shown to have a positive effect on the brain: "Overall, participants who ranked high on the healthy diet scale did better on ten tests of memory than those with lower diet scores. *The same held true for those who took in more caffeine*" (emphasis added).[29] It should be noted, however, that not all studies have shown these same beneficial effects for consumption of caffeine.

And finally, a study on rats that was conducted by Fernando Gomez-Pinilla at the David Geffen School of Medicine at UCLA and published in the *Journal of Physiology* showed how a diet high in fructose negatively affects brain function, and how omega-3 fatty acids can help to minimize those effects. Gomez-Pinilla reported, "Our findings illustrate that what you eat affects how you think. . . . Eating a high-fructose diet over the long term alters your brain's ability to learn and remember information. But adding omega-3 fatty acids to your meals can help minimize the damage."[30]

Gomez-Pinilla says, "DHA [a form of omega-3 fatty acid found mainly in oily fish but also in nuts, seeds, whole grains, and dark green leafy vegetables] is essential for synaptic function—brain cells' ability to transmit signals to one another. This is the mechanism that makes learning and memory possible."

Although the detrimental health effects of high-fructose corn syrup have been receiving increased attention lately, Americans are still consuming too much of the sweetener—about thirty-five pounds per capita according to the United States Department of Agriculture—mainly in commercial baked goods and soft drinks.

These are just a few of the many studies that have linked nutrition to brain function over the past several years. Unfortunately, brain buddies Einstein and Gödel didn't have the access we have now to the knowledge derived from these scientific advances. So, even with full knowledge of the brilliant work they accomplished in their lifetimes, one can't help speculating as to whether such information might not have allowed them to do even more.

Fortunately, we are now privy to about a half century's worth of additional scientific research into the link between nutrition and brain health. While I'm certainly not suggesting that using this knowledge in conjunction with what we now know about the contributions of exercise and overall fitness to maximum brain function will turn you into an Einstein or a Gödel, I do know that following the ReSYNC Method, which is based on that knowledge, will allow you to become the smartest you that you can possibly be.

So what are the best foods you can eat regularly to avoid Alzheimer's disease and keep your brain working to the max? Here's a list of the top eight:

1. **Apples.** The peel contains quercetin, an antioxidant that supports brain function and a healthy nervous system—so eat your apples with the peel.

2. **Berries.** All kinds of berries are rich in vitamin C and contain a number of antioxidants that help to reduce inflammation and the harmful effects of free radicals.

3. **Concord grape juice.** Concord grapes contain polyphenols, a type of antioxidant that has been shown to improve cognition with aging. One study showed that older adults with mild cognitive impairment did better on tests of neurocognitive function after consuming Concord grape juice for sixteen weeks than the control group, who were given a placebo.[31]

4. **Curry powder.** Curcumin (turmeric), an ancient Indian spice found in curry powder, is an antioxidant and anti-inflammatory that may help to reduce the risk of developing Alzheimer's disease in several ways, including the reduction in formation of the plaques in the brain that characterize the illness.[32] Curcumin is most effective when consumed with a small amount of black pepper.

5. **Dark chocolate.** Research out of Harvard Medical School has shown that people who drank two cups of cocoa a day had improved memory and blood flow to the brain.[33] But it has to be really dark chocolate that contains significant amounts of flavonoids that are good for the brain. And don't overdo, because even the healthiest of chocolate is high in calories.

6. **Fatty fish.** Fish such as salmon and mackerel are high in omega-3 fatty acids, which are known to have multiple health benefits and have been shown to protect against a variety of mental disorders, including dementia.[34]

7. **Leafy greens.** We know that all kinds of leafy greens contain vitamins and minerals that protect us from the effects of aging and a variety of diseases—which include diseases of the brain.

8. **Nuts.** All kinds—from almonds to walnuts to hazelnuts—contain omega-3 fatty acids that, like the omega-3s in fatty fish, help protect and improve brain function.

ReSYNCING Your Body and Brain

If I've been doing my job right, it should be clear by now that whatever helps improve your body also improves your brain—and vice versa.

As you start to learn the exercises I describe in chapter 2, you will be using many different muscles and muscle groups simultaneously, and your brain will have to figure out how to do that. Once you accomplish your goal, your brain, too, will have reached a new level of fitness, and you can then use that increased brainpower to carry out the next new task you need to complete. Power in one area leads to power in another.

So, if you're exercising, and at the same time you're eating a diet based on saturated fats, as in steak and fried chicken, you're going to feel terrible, because you're muscles need good, clean fats to function properly. What's going to happen then is that your brain will tell you to change your diet, and when you do that, your body and your brain will be working together to create overall health.

Knowledge does not exist in a vacuum. Whatever information or expertise you acquire in one area of your life can and should be applied to your life as a whole. That is the yellow brick road that will lead you to becoming the person you were always meant to be.

Twenty-Eight Tips to Boost Your Brainpower

1. **Turn off the TV.** We all know that being a couch potato isn't good for our physical health, but a study published in the *American Journal of Preventive Medicine* has also shown that watching excessive amounts of television has been associated with a lower quality of mental health.[35] In another study, researchers followed 3,247 adults over the course of twenty-five years and found that those who watched the most television did worse on one or more cognitive tests, and those with low physical activity performed poorly on one of the tests. The odds of poor cognitive function were almost twice as high among people with both—that is, high levels of TV viewing *and* low levels of physical activity.[36]

2. **Read a novel just for the fun of it.** Researchers at Stanford University have found that reading for pleasure (in this case, Jane Austen's *Mansfield Park)* affected different parts of the brain from those associated with reading as a learning task.[37] Many studies have looked at the way reading fiction affects the brain. One in particular, done at Emory University and published in the journal *Brain Connectivity,* found that

after reading a specific novel, students' brains showed increases in both connectivity and function. Gregory Berns, who led the study, noted, "The fact that we're detecting [neural changes] over a few days for a randomly assigned novel suggests that your favorite novels could certainly have a bigger and longer-lasting effect on the biology of your brain."[38]

3. **Play a board game.** Whether it's Monopoly or Scrabble or some other game of your choice, board games require strategizing, which challenges your brain to work harder.

4. **Memorize a poem.** Can't remember where you put your keys? The name of your best friend's sister? Why you're standing in front of the open refrigerator? Memory is one of the first things to fail us as we age. By memorizing something new, like a poem, we help to keep our memory sharper.

5. **Get out of your comfort zone.** Trying an activity you've never done before forces your brain to work harder. Just as physical exercise tones your muscles, mental exercise hones your mental skills.[39]

6. **Take a chess lesson.** Chess is a game that requires you to plan ahead and anticipate moves your opponent is likely to make. If you're just starting out, this could be difficult—which is good, because it forces you to use your brain to solve problems in a new way.

7. **Play a game of Ping-Pong.** Ping-Pong improves hand-eye coordination and sharpens reflexes at the same time as it burns calories and provides an opportunity for social interaction.

8. **Match the color to your task.** Science has shown that color may affect your ability to succeed at different kinds of tasks. If you're trying to complete a detail-oriented task, try to surround yourself with red. If you need to ramp up creativity, put yourself in a blue environment.[40]

9. **Try a new recipe.** Take a look at the list of foods on pages 110–111 that help you focus. Choose one and make a new recipe using that food.

10. **Try googling.** A study published in the *American Journal of Geriatric Psychiatry* has suggested that over time, surfing the Internet "may alter the brain's responsiveness in neural circuits controlling decision making and complex reasoning."[41] What this means is that searching online may activate parts of the brain that would not be used if you were reading a printed text. So don't let anyone tell you all that Internet surfing is just a waste of time.

11. **Jump rope.** According to a 2009 Swedish study, it's good for your heart and your brain. Jumping rope is an aerobic activity that gets your heart pumping, and the study showed that cardiovascular fitness can raise your verbal intelligence by 50 percent. "Increased cardiovascular fitness . . . was associated with better cognitive scores," says Maria Aberg, who led the study. "In contrast, muscular strength [was] only weakly associated with . . . intelligence."[42]

12. **Play a video game.** No, I'm not kidding! A recent study done at the University of Rochester confirmed a link between first-person video games and enhanced visual awareness in the "real" world, which is a crucial building block for IQ. A first-person video game is one in which the player experiences the action from the point of view of the virtual protagonist.[43]

13. **Go to the zoo.** You'll be outdoors, which is certainly good for your physical and mental health. While you're there, read the information posted near the enclosures about the various animals. You'll learn something while you're having a good time.

14. **Visit your local farmers' market.** Look for the fresh fruits and berries listed on page 203 and give yourself a delicious treat that will also increase your brainpower. You'll know your food is really fresh, and you'll also be showing your support for local growers.

15. **Relax with aromatherapy.** Either inhaling or massaging with essential

oils can help you relax and reduce stress, which in turn allows your brain to refocus and concentrate on whatever it is you need or want to accomplish. Among the many essential oils available, lavender and chamomile are among those used most often to promote relaxation.[44]

16. **Get out your binoculars and go bird-watching.** Yes, it's relaxing and a great source of exercise, but it also requires mental alertness. A bird can fly away in the blink of an eye, so you need to keep your eyes open and your attention focused—at least if you really want to see anything.

17. **Play pool.** You'd be amazed by how much mental focus goes into a simple game of pool. You need to figure angles, have good hand-eye coordination, and use your problem-solving skills. And all the while you are also practicing balance, becoming more flexible, and toning various muscles.

18. **Change your daily routine.** Take a different route to work, or go to a new restaurant for lunch and order a food you've never tried before. You'll be making your brain work a bit harder and creating new connections.

19. **Force yourself to focus.** Find a painting with many different colors (you can probably do this on your computer), and make yourself focus on seeing only one color at a time.

20. **Count backward.** Start at 100 and count backward to 1 to make your brain work in a new way.

21. **Visualize your living space.** Close your eyes and visualize the room you're in. Include as many small details as possible.

22. **Take a trip through time.** Sit down with a pen and paper and write down the addresses and telephone numbers of every place you've lived in their proper order, starting with the oldest.

23. **Write with your nondominant hand.** Find a passage on a subject

that interests you, and copy it, using pen and paper, with your non-dominant hand.

24. **Read backward.** Find an article on health and fitness, and read it from end to beginning. When you're done, see how much you can remember of what you've read.

25. **Do a jigsaw puzzle.** Instead of laying out the pieces picture-side-up, spread them out with only the backs showing so you have to solve the puzzle using just the shapes.

26. **Try to remember telephone numbers.** Remembering phone numbers is something no one needs to do anymore because they're all stored in our phones. Sit down with a pad and pen, and see how many of your friends' and family members' phone numbers you can recall.

27. **Listen to classical music.** A study has shown that listening to twenty minutes of classical music positively affected genes involved in dopamine secretion and transport, synaptic function, learning, and memory.[45]

28. **Laugh at a joke.** According to neurologist Richard Restak, humor is associated with "brain networks involving the temporal and frontal lobes in the cerebral cortex. Located near the top of the brain, these cortical areas are related to speech, general information, and the appreciation of contradiction and illogicality."[46]

CHAPTER 5

ReSYNC Your Spirit: Twenty-Eight Days to Spiritual Balance

Body, mind, and spirit compose the holy health trinity; any one or two without the others will not provide total health.

We have already discussed the roles played by exercise and diet, and in chapter 4 we talked about how fitness can affect the brain as well as how the brain itself contributes to overall health. Now it's time to add the all-important spiritual component of the ReSYNC program. Many people find that once their bodies become healthier, their spirituality also begins to flourish.

Introducing Fitness to Churchgoers

To me, it has always been perfectly clear that whatever affects one area of your life affects your life as a whole. You can't separate your brain from your heart or your body from your spirit.

When I started working with members of churches, however, I found that many people did not make this connection among body, mind, and spirit. In fact, they didn't really understand why a church would want or need to have a fitness program at all. To them, church was about the spiritual, not the physical. "What does this have to do with faith?" they asked me. I realized right away that I wasn't going to be able to teach fitness to people at church the same way I had been teaching it in a gym.

People go to a gym specifically to work out; they go because they're motivated. In a church, however, I discovered that I needed a way to open the minds of my new (and reluctant) clients. The way I did that was first to remind them that they actually went to church for many different reasons. "You go to church to worship. You even go to eat," I said. "You go to listen to music. So why not go to church to get fit? Your church is your community; why not work with one another to improve your physical health?" I convinced at least a few of them to give it a try.

Before and After

Based on my own experience and what I constantly hear from others, Americans are driven by the need to do everything faster, better, sooner. We are afraid that if we stop for a moment, we will be left behind, and because of that, we don't give ourselves a chance to breathe.

That was certainly true for a lot of the people I was working with at Lakewood Church. Like many Americans, they led very stressful lives. They got up, went to work, came home, and were too tired to do much else. For some, life was monotonous, the same day in and day out, except perhaps for the week or two they went on vacation.

When I started the fitness program at the church, much of the congregation was out of shape and overweight. They said they had very little energy to do much more than work; they couldn't even focus on participating in church activities or on increasing their faith.

Then, as they began to work with me, they started getting fitter, and even if they hadn't lost weight, they felt better. Soon their lives had changed. They became more spiritually active. They were thinking about the actual meaning of the biblical verses they'd been reading for years. As I've learned, the fitter people are, the more energy they have to devote to their spiritual life.

When you start to exercise, you feel better in the mornings. You may be a little achy, but it's a good ache, a soreness that comes from having worked out the day before. You have more energy. You go to work and you aren't so tired afterward. Soon you are eating better, too, because a healthy body rebels against unhealthy food; the foods you used to love now make you feel sick. You feel more refreshed.

About two or three months after members of our congregation began the ReSYNC program, they were standing up straighter and singing in church with a stronger voice. Their fellow churchgoers noticed the difference, and they, too, joined the program. They began to encourage one another, and they lifted one another up as a church community. Because their friends, neighbors, and family members also saw how much happier and more fulfilled they had become, more and more of them began coming to our church to see what the ReSYNC Method was all about. As a result, hundreds more people have now joined, and they, too, are enjoying the benefits that come from introducing physical fitness into a Christian community.

By changing yourself, you change the people around you, and your whole life changes for the better.

Making the Christian Connection

When I began the fitness program at Lakewood Church, I realized that to convince my fitness flock to follow me, I would have to provide them with biblical examples and points of reference that would resonate with them. Doing that turned out to be a lot easier than I thought it might be.

The world's largest religions advocate for health and fitness. The followers want to live in a way that most closely emulates their leader. For Christians, that is following in Jesus' footsteps, which, for many who are used to being sedentary and out of shape, is easier said than done. In fact, many people were—and continue to be—surprised when I point out that in addition to his spiritual guidance, Jesus had much to teach us about leading a healthy lifestyle.

Don Colbert, author of *The Seven Pillars of Health*, estimates that Jesus walked at least twenty-one thousand miles in his lifetime, which equates to more than twenty miles every day. And that was in the desert, where it was incredibly hot in the summer and incredibly cold in the winter.[1]

To put this number in perspective, consider how many miles the average American walks in a day. According to various sources, it is between 5,000 and 6,000 steps, or between two and a half and three miles. According to the Centers for Disease Control, we should be averaging between 7,000 and 8,000 steps (or between three and a half and four miles) a day,[2] although I believe that to be healthy we should be walking at least 10,000 steps (about five miles) every day. In some countries, such as Australia and Switzerland, people are averaging about 9,500 steps a day.[3]

Based on those numbers, Jesus walked about eight times more than the average American. In addition to being a great form of exercise that is available to virtually everyone, walking has been shown to strengthen joints, combat stress and depression, contribute to heart health, and lower blood pressure—to name just a few of the many reasons I recommend that you walk as much as possible.

Jesus also followed what was then, and would be even today, an extremely healthy diet. Many scientists and historians examined what foods, in addition to those actually mentioned in the Bible, would have been available to Jesus during his lifetime, and they have concluded that he would have been eating an organic, primarily plant-based diet composed mainly of whole grains, lentils, chickpeas, herbs and spices, fruits (including figs, dates, grapes, apples, and watermelons), vegetables (including onions and garlic), nuts and seeds, as well as fish and lean meat.[4]

As a poor, itinerant carpenter, Jesus probably did not have access to large quantities of food on a regular basis, so it would be safe to assume that he probably wasn't overeating! When food was plentiful, he might have eaten more, but there surely would also have been times when food was scarce. In any case, during biblical times, people didn't have access to unlimited quantities and varieties of foods at every hour of the day and night, as we do today.

Going back about thirteen hundred years, we see that Moses led by example. To escape captivity in Egypt, he and his people, the Israelites, walked through the desert for forty years. He climbed Mount Sinai not once but twice, and then he carried two big stone tablets with the Ten Commandments on them back down the mountain. Chronologically, Moses was an old man by then, but physically and spiritually he was much younger, and he had a higher purpose to drive him on.

Muslims follow the prophet Muhammad, who advocated eating slowly, which would also lead to eating less, for better digestion and health. He was also a strong proponent of physical exercise and urged parents to teach their children swimming, horseback riding, and archery.[5]

Turning to Buddhism, we learn that Siddhartha Gautama, the prince who is generally accepted as the founder of Buddhism, was trained to be a warrior and a leader of men in defense of his people in Nepal. His father, Suddhodana, is said to have been a skilled swordsman who won many battles.[6] Given what is known (or at least universally accepted) about his actual life, why is the Buddha generally depicted as a jolly, smiling fat man with a big belly? As it turns out, that's not Siddhartha at all. It's a case of mistaken identity. The "fat" or "laughing" Buddha first appeared in China. But that guy is actually Budai, a deity in Chinese folklore, whose identity somehow became conflated or confused with that of Siddhartha.[7]

Other contemporary images, religious and otherwise, have evolved into false representations. Take, for example, the beloved Christmas character we call Santa Claus, or Saint Nick. The "real" Saint Nicholas was actually a bishop who lived in the fourth century in what is now Turkey. He was apparently a kind and generous man born into a wealthy family who helped the poor by giving them secret gifts. Because of his kindness and good deeds, he was made a saint, but later he was exiled and put in prison by the emperor Diocletian.[8] After the reformation in sixteenth-century Europe, stories about Saint Nicholas fell out of favor, but someone still had to deliver secret gifts to children on Christmas. That's when the legend of Santa Claus was born.

All the images we see of the original Saint Nicholas are of a tall, slim man, not a jolly fat man in a red suit. That image apparently evolved over a period of about twenty years, starting in the late 1860s, when the artist Thomas Nast began drawing Santa for the magazine *Harper's Weekly*. The red suit, which many people attribute to the influence of Coca-Cola, is actually a reference to the bishop's robes worn by the original Saint Nicholas. How his belly developed we don't know, but it seems that big bellies are generally associated with good humor and generosity—despite what we now know about the many health issues related to obesity.[9]

Reconnecting Body and Spirit

Unfortunately, it appears to be the Christian community that has fallen the farthest from the physical ideals modeled by their spiritual leader. According to a study done by Krista C. Cline and Kenneth F. Ferraro at Purdue University, the Christian community is the most overweight religious group in the United States—with anywhere from 17 to 30 percent being obese, depending on denomination—compared to Jews at 1 percent and Buddhists and Hindus at 0.7 percent.[10]

It doesn't have to be that way. Yes, there are temptations all around us every day. We almost never have to walk anywhere anymore; we have machines to do the work that our ancestors would have had to do by hand; we have so many tasty food choices that we could easily (and often do) eat ourselves into oblivion. But the other side of that coin is that we have unprecedented access to scientific knowledge about the value of various types of exercise and the nutritional content of every type of food. We know what lifestyle changes we can make to remain healthier and happier throughout our lives. Ignorance is no longer a valid excuse. Among the many things science has taught us about the link between physical fitness and spirituality, several studies have shown that exercise can increase levels of the hormones dopamine and serotonin in the blood and the brain. Both of these neurochemicals help to elevate mood and reduce feelings of pain and stress. These physical changes directly enhance our sense of well-being.[11]

Exercise—and particularly aerobic exercise—has also been shown to reduce levels of cortisol, known as the stress hormone, in the blood.[12] All of these chemical changes, brought on by exercise, make us feel alive in a way that many say they haven't experienced before.

In addition to regular exercise, eating nutritious foods that boost your mood is the other vital component of achieving physical and spiritual well-being.

Not surprisingly, it turns out that many of the foods we should be eating are those that Jesus probably ate—including fish and seafood, lean meats, nuts and seeds, whole grains, and beans.[13]

When you are well nourished, less stressed, and feeling good about yourself and the world, it stands to reason that you will be more likely to engage in activities that lift your spirit and increase spirituality. When you feel strong, when you think you can move a mountain, you can move a mountain. When you say you are open to receiving greatness, you will then receive it. I have seen these changes in hundreds of people using the ReSYNC Method.

Community Ups Your Spiritual Ante

Studies have shown that in addition to exercise and proper nutrition, having a close-knit group of family and friends can help reduce stress and protect us from disease.[14]

One way to achieve that sense of support is by belonging to some kind of spiritual community. I see this all the time as I work with church groups whose members are supportive of the efforts being made by their fellow congregants, but there is also scientific evidence to confirm my personal observations.

For example, a survey of health attitudes conducted by the Robert Wood Johnson Foundation in 2015 found that people who do not feel strongly connected to a community are less likely than those who do to engage in health-promoting behaviors or to work with others for positive change.[15]

Another study, by Chaeyoon Lim and Robert D. Putnam, found that religious service attendance, and in particular the friendships people built through participation in a religious congregation, correlated with a greater sense of life satisfaction when compared to people who did not have those connections.[16] Taken together, what these studies mean to me is that people who have a strong sense of community—in my case, specifically a Christian community—gain emotional strength and an increased sense of well-being, which also correlate with a longer and healthier life.

In addition, a study by Laura D. Kubzansky and Rebecca C. Thurston followed 6,265 men and women aged twenty-five to seventy-four who, at the beginning of the study, did not have coronary heart disease (CHD). At the end of the fifteen-year follow-up, the researchers determined that those who expressed the highest levels of emotional vitality (characterized by a sense of energy, positive well-being, and effective emotion regulation) had a significantly reduced risk of CHD when compared with those who expressed the lowest levels, leading them to hypothesize that emotional vitality reduces the risk of heart disease.[17]

So, if being fitter and healthier allows us to become more spiritual, it is also true that having robust emotional strength and strong spiritual ties makes us more physically fit.

But community is only half the equation. To have a truly vibrant sense of spiritual well-being, we also need to take some quiet time alone, get in touch with what is truly important in life, and reconnect with our spirituality.

One of the oldest and most global of spiritual practices is meditation. The Bible mentions meditation many times,[18] and according to the World Community for Christian Meditation, "We meditate in order to take the attention off ourselves. (Jesus said to leave self behind.) In the Christian tradition, contemplation is seen as a grace and as a reciprocal work of love. Not surprisingly, then, if we find that we become more loving people as a result of meditating, this will express itself in all our relationships, our work, and our sense of service especially to those in any kind of need."[19]

In *Satisfy Your Soul*, Bruce Demarest, professor of Christian formation at Denver Seminary in Littleton, Colorado, wrote, "A quieted heart is our best preparation for all this work of God. . . . Meditation refocuses us from ourselves and from the world so that we reflect on God's Word, His nature, His abilities, and His works. . . . So we prayerfully ponder, muse, and 'chew' the words of Scripture. . . . The goal is simply to permit the Holy Spirit to activate the life-giving Word of God."[20]

So, if meditation increases spirituality, how does it contribute to our health? Meditation takes our attention off ourselves, which in turn reduces stress and anxiety and lowers our heart rate and blood pressure. If we are less stressed mentally and physically, it follows that we will be happier and healthier.

A 2014 study by Perla Kaliman and colleagues at the Institute of Biomedical Research of Barcelona, Spain, showed that mindful meditation can lead to alterations in the expression of genes, including inflammatory genes that help to speed physical recovery from stress.[21]

According to Kaliman, "the changes were observed in genes that are the current targets of anti-inflammatory and analgesic drugs." It would seem, therefore, that meditation could have curative effects similar to those of medication.[22]

In chapter 1 we discussed a study indicating that people who placed more importance on religion and spirituality showed a thicker cortex than those who did not. Another study, by Eileen Luders and colleagues at the UCLA School of Medicine and the University of Jena (Germany), showed other cortical differences between longtime meditators and those who did not meditate, indicating that the meditators might be better at controlling daydreaming and mind wandering—in other words, they might be better able to stay focused. The researchers hypothesize that since the observed cortical changes are related to human behavioral traits, "the observed alterations in long-term practitioners might reflect specific traits associated with meditation (that is, higher levels of introspection, awareness, response control, compassion, etc.)."[23] And, I would add, they might also reflect the patience and focus to follow aspects of the ReSYNC plan that contribute to fitness and health.

Reawakening Your Spirit

The ReSYNC Method helps you reawaken the spirit that may have been dormant in your life, and once that spark is lit, you will have the energy and the commitment to increase the spirituality that gives a deeper meaning to everything you do. Over and over again it has been shown that increased spirituality leads to all-around better health and greater happiness. It is a virtuous cycle.

The ReSYNC Method is all about feeling more alive. My goal for you is to start each day with a positive spirit. Wake up in the morning filled with energy, look in the mirror and smile, drink a big glass of water, and have a healthy breakfast that will energize you. Enjoy your ride to work listening to music you love, and be a positive force at your workplace.

Be the sun that gives energy to those around you. Be a loving spouse, parent, sibling, and child. Be a supportive friend and coworker; focus on the positive in people, and realize that we all make mistakes.

You will achieve all this, but it will be a journey. Like anything that is worthwhile, it isn't going to happen overnight. It will require patience and perseverance.

I can't tell you how many people have come up to me at the very beginning of their journey to total health and complained that they didn't feel any different. If that's how you feel, I'm not surprised. But just think about this: Have you ever slept for ten to twelve hours and felt even more tired when you woke up? Maybe it took you an hour or so before you could function properly. That's because of the muscle atrophy created by lack of movement and dehydration while you were sleeping. Now think about how long you've let your spirit sleep—it could be five, ten, or even fifteen years. No wonder you won't feel the full effect of the ReSYNC Method in one day!

And remember, even the Almighty took six days to create the heavens and the earth. It didn't happen overnight. But the journey you're about to begin, I promise you, will be well worth the effort. You will experience the reawakening of your spirit, and in the end, you will enjoy a deeper, more spiritually satisfying connection to the Divine.

Twenty-Eight Tips to ReSync Your Spirit and Uplift Your Life

1. **Build yourself up.** Find three things about yourself to appreciate. Generally speaking, we're really good at tearing ourselves down. Today, make it your goal to find three qualities in yourself for which you deserve a pat on the back.

2. **Talk to a stranger.** According to social scientist Elizabeth Dunn, we tend to be pleasant and "put on a happy face" when we interact with a stranger, and we then tend to carry over that positive mood to subsequent interactions with our friends and family.[24]

3. **Try something new.** Trying new things can improve your cognition and social skills. Do one thing today that takes you outside your comfort zone. If you make this a regular practice, you will learn to overcome your fears, build your strengths, have fun, and challenge yourself.[25]

4. **Overcome procrastination and accomplish one goal.** When you stop procrastinating and actually do something you've been avoiding, you'll lift your spirit and feel better about yourself.[26]

5. **Unplug from unnecessary information.** Just for a day, turn off

your smartphone, your tablet, and your computer. Removing yourself from all the mostly unnecessary information coming your way 24/7 will allow you to clear your mind and focus on what really makes you happy.

6. **Learn one new thing.** Maybe there's something you've always wondered about but never took the time to research. Learning something new will give you a sense of accomplishment and increase your self-esteem.

7. **Take a hike.** Yes, literally. Studies have shown that simply being outdoors makes us happy.[27]

8. **Smile!** Studies show that when we smile we actually feel better, even if we weren't feeling so great in the first place.[28]

9. **Try one new mood-boosting food today.** Look at the list on pages 201–208, and choose one food you haven't tried before. If you don't like it, you can always try another one on another day. By doing this regularly, you will slowly build your repertoire of mood-boosting foods in your regular diet.

10. **Play with a pet.** A few minutes petting a cat or dog has been shown to increase levels of serotonin, which is related to feelings of well-being, and oxytocin, known as the "hug hormone." In addition, petting a dog or cat will decrease levels of cortisol, the stress hormone that also regulates appetite and cravings for carbohydrates.[29]

11. **Dance.** Whatever the style, whether alone or with a partner, dancing not only improves physical fitness but also helps elevate your mood. It's hard to remain stressed or depressed when you're dancing.[30]

12. **Stand up straight.** Research has shown that an expansive, open posture helps you to feel more powerful and actually reduces levels of the stress hormone cortisol in your body.[31]

13. **Remind yourself of what's important.** Take time to think about

what's really important in your life. Doing that will help you get past the little annoyances we all experience and concentrate on the good things coming your way.

14. **Do something you love.** It should be obvious—to raise your spirit do something that makes you happy. But too many of us are so busy trying to do everything we *have* to do that we forget to do the things we love.

15. **Give yourself a break today.** These days everyone is so concerned with "keeping up" that we never take a day off. Declare that today is a vacation day. You'll find that the world doesn't come to an end, and when you go back to your regular job or routine the next day, you'll be more energized and better able to complete whatever it is you need to do.

16. **Pat yourself on the back.** Think of something you've accomplished—it could be anything from losing five pounds (or more, or less) to finishing a task you've been avoiding—and give yourself a reward, even if it's no more than a simple, and literal, pat on the back. Acknowledging your accomplishment will make you feel better about yourself, lift your spirits, and make it more likely that it becomes a lifelong habit.[32]

17. **Phone a friend.** Maintaining a sense of connection and community is essential for our spiritual well-being, but finding the time to keep up with friends and family can be difficult. Make it your goal to call someone with whom you may have lost touch, and reignite the spark that may have been in danger of dying.

18. **Look in the mirror and love yourself today.** Very often when we look in the mirror, all we see are flaws. We compare ourselves to the unrealistic standards presented by the media every day of our lives. Today, when you look in the mirror, notice and acknowledge all the good things you see. Be happy with who you are.

19. **Perform an act of kindness.** Whether it's helping a stranger cross a busy street or helping a colleague complete an assignment, performing an act of kindness, no matter how small, will lift your spirits and elevate your mood for the rest of the day.

20. **Sing a song.** Singing has been found to boost your mood and may also help to increase antibodies that fight disease, so by all means, sing a song to lift your spirit and enhance your physical well-being. If you're shy, sing in the shower at the top of your lungs![33]

21. **Take time to be grateful.** Actually taking the time to write down the things for which you are grateful will help you look on the bright side of life and be happy for what you have.[34]

22. **Hug someone.** Hugging, cuddling, and even hand-holding increase levels of oxytocin, the bonding and feel-good hormone, in your blood.[35]

23. **Have a good laugh.** Laughing allows you to take in more oxygen-rich air and increases the endorphins that are released by your brain.[36] Being with someone who is filled with laughter makes you happier as well. It's hard to be down and depressed when you're surrounded by joy.

24. **Buy a new novel.** Or borrow one—and start to read it. Reading fiction can create greater empathy as you become emotionally involved in the lives of the characters, which can then translate into your making better connections with people in your own life.[37]

25. **Visit a museum or an art gallery.** Aside from the religious subjects prevalent in medieval and Renaissance art, viewing art of all types, including the modern and the abstract, has a soothing and uplifting effect on the heart and the soul.[38]

26. **Take a yoga class.** Yoga helps quiet your thoughts, lower blood pressure, reduce anxiety, and in general, puts you in a more spiritual frame of mind.[39]

27. **Put on an outfit you love.** How we dress often reflects how we feel.

So, to boost your spirits, put on something that makes you happy and feel good about yourself when you look in the mirror.[40]

28. **Volunteer.** Find a cause or an event you believe in, and volunteer your time, even if it's only for a few hours or a day. You will probably find that the happiness you get from helping will make you want to do it again and again.[41]

CHAPTER 6

Putting It All Together

At this point, you've learned what you need to do to ReSYNC your fitness. You have a diet plan to lose those extra pounds. You have my twenty-eight suggestions for boosting your brainpower and an additional twenty-eight suggestions for becoming more spiritual. Now is the time to put those four components of the ReSYNC Method together and get started. Don't fear. It's not complicated. You just need to follow a few simple rules:

- Make sure the meals and snacks you choose are appropriate for the week you're in. In other words, don't choose foods from week three if you're still in week two.
- Determine your level of fitness and choose an appropriate exercise program for each day.
- Make sure you stick to the portion quantities stated in the diet plan.

- It's okay to repeat meals and snacks if you find you enjoy some more than others, but try to get as much variety as possible into your diet.
- Do at least one thing to boost your brain each day.
- Implement at least one tip for increasing your spirituality every day.

I want to give you as much freedom of choice as possible within the parameters we've established, so you're going to be making your own food, exercise, spirituality, and brain booster choices. But you also need to stick with the program, which means that you need to keep track of what you're doing. Therefore I'm providing you with a kind of journal in the form of a chart to fill in for each of the twenty-eight days of the ReSYNC Method program (see page 173).

You can fill it in as far in advance as you want—for example, maybe you'd like to do a week at a time so that you can shop for the week's groceries, knowing you'll have the foods you need on hand, and can plan your days in advance to make time for your workout as well as your spiritual and brain booster practices.

Maybe you know that on a particular day you'll be eating dinner out, so you can plan the rest of your day, including your diet, around that.

Whatever works for you is okay as long as you fill in your chart every day. You can write in the book (I give you permission to do that), or you can copy the pages into a notebook or onto single sheets of paper.

In the end, you're on the honor system here, but if you cheat, the only one you'll be cheating is yourself.

CHAPTER 7

The Power of ReSYNCing for Life

From the earliest of times, humans have been seeking some magical means of turning back the clock and beating death. From Shangri-La to the Fountain of Youth, we keep hoping to discover the secret to eternal life. Who among us would not want to live longer, look younger, and be healthier?

Interestingly enough, in biblical times, many great patriarchs lived to ages that would be unimaginable today. As the Bible tells us in Genesis 5 (NIV):

> After Seth was born, Adam lived 800 years. . . . Altogether, Adam lived a total of 930 years. (vv. 4–5)
>
> After he became the father of Enosh, Seth lived 807 years. . . . Altogether, Seth lived a total of 912 years. (vv. 7–8)
>
> After he became the father of Kenan, Enosh lived 815 years. . . . Altogether, Enosh lived a total of 905 years. (vv. 10–11).

Then, skipping a few long-lived generations:

> After he became the father of Methuselah, Enoch walked faithfully
> with God 300 years. . . . Altogether, Enoch lived a total of 365 years.
> (vv. 22–23)
> After he became the father of Lamech, Methuselah lived 782
> years. . . . Altogether, Methuselah lived a total of 969 years.
> (vv. 26–27)
> When Lamech had lived 182 years, he had a son. He named him
> Noah. . . . Altogether, Lamech lived a total of 777 years, and then
> he died. (vv. 28–31)

Somewhere along the way, however, it seems that God became angry with
what he had created:

> The LORD said, "My Spirit will not contend with humans forever, for they are
> mortal; their days will be *a hundred and twenty years*" (Genesis 6:3 NIV, empha-
> sis added)

Why Has Our Life Span Been Shortened?

Admittedly, 120 is a ripe old age. The oldest person in modern times whose
age has been officially documented was Jeanne Calment, a Frenchwoman who
died in 1997 at the age of 122.[1] But why are we now living much shorter lives
than those recorded up to the time of this woman's death?

Some people would say we're paying for Adam's original sin as well as the
subsequent sins of humanity that caused God to destroy all of humankind
except for Noah and his family. Let's think about that. If God created Adam in

his image, Adam must have been an almost perfect specimen of man, and the Bible tells us that he lived in a perfect environment:

> The LORD God had planted a garden in the east, in Eden; and there he put the man he had formed. The LORD God made all kinds of trees grow out of the ground—trees that were pleasing to the eye and good for food. In the middle of the garden were the tree of life and the tree of the knowledge of good and evil. (Genesis 2:8–9 NIV)

So, yes, it is possible to say that had Adam not eaten the forbidden fruit, we all might still be living in a perfect environment and enjoying the food from all those other trees God planted instead of growing fatter and reducing our life expectancy with double cheeseburgers and crispy fried chicken. But it doesn't have to be that way.

The problem is that by seeking a magical reprieve such as the mythical Fountain of Youth, we're going about it the wrong way. We may not be able to live forever, but science has shown us that we *can* live much longer than most of us do. In fact, life expectancy is on the rise. And I've also seen for myself that people can remain healthy—or even become healthier—late in life.

Two of my most memorable older clients came to me from opposite ends of the health spectrum.

I met Arthur in 2002, shortly after I arrived in the States. I noticed him in the gym because he was so fit, and I was shocked to learn that he was eighty-seven. Based on the way he walked, the way he held himself, and the way he talked, he seemed more like someone in his fifties. The only clue to his true age was that he obviously was coloring his hair.

Arthur told me that he'd joined the first gym to open in his area back in the 1940s, shortly after the end of World War II, and had been working out once a day, five to six days a week, ever since. Back then, he said, his friends thought he was crazy. People only worked out if they were boxers or athletes; no one worked out just to be healthy. But Arthur had been following a healthy lifestyle, including his diet, all of his life. Of course, he said, when he was a young man, there weren't so many processed foods available, so there weren't as many unhealthy choices as we have today. Still, I was impressed.

After I moved to another location, I lost touch with Arthur. Then, in 2015, I was having dinner in a restaurant when I saw a large group at a nearby table. The waiter told me it was a birthday celebration for someone who was turning one hundred years old. I was intrigued; I had to see this guy. I made my way over to the table and noticed someone in the group who looked familiar; I just couldn't place him. I thought maybe I'd seen him on television. But he obviously knew me, because he waved me over and greeted me by name. At that moment, I realized he was Arthur. He looked exactly the same except for the fact that he no longer colored his hair. He was still vibrant and in great shape, and he told me that he was still working out every day. That was the first time I really knew that you could be one hundred years old and fit. It is a reality!

When Margaret first came to me, she was at the opposite end of the health spectrum. Born in England, she had come to the States when she was a young girl. Now seventy-eight, Margaret had more or less lost her zest for life. She said that she just wasn't enjoying herself anymore, and her daughter had brought her to me to see if I could help her.

That first day we just talked and walked a bit outdoors. Margaret said she wanted to go out because she almost never left her house. But she also got out of breath very quickly, so we had to stop frequently, and after a short while she said she wanted to go back inside because she was in pain. I was actually having a hard time trying to figure out how I could motivate her to help herself so she would feel better. I gave myself a month to see what I could do.

Margaret said she woke up at half past four every morning no matter what time she went to bed, and she ate only once a day because she was never hungry. The first thing I asked her to do was just to drink three glasses of water a day, but she said she wasn't thirsty and she didn't like water. So I asked what flavors she liked, and she told me strawberry. I asked her daughter to buy some strawberries and put them through a blender with some water to make flavored water.

The next time Margaret came to me, she told me that she'd actually been drinking four glasses of water every day (one more than I had asked for) because she liked the strawberry taste so much. And she told me that she already felt more alert and had more energy. Now she was getting into this and asked me if there was something else I could suggest for her to do. I said, "Yes, just go over to that wall and push against it with as much strength as you have." Of course, she didn't have much, so she pushed against the wall for about five seconds, and I could tell her muscles were giving out. She did that maybe fifteen or twenty times during the hour we were together, so the entire workout amounted to fewer than two minutes.

Next, I asked her to eat one green apple a day. She said she didn't like green apples, but there was one variety of red apple she liked, so I said that was fine, so long as she had one every day. I also asked her to drink one more glass of water a day.

The next step was to get her to eat more protein. Margaret wasn't eating any meat, so I asked her to add a piece of fish to her diet—any kind she liked, just one piece every day.

One week at a time, I slowly increased her protein intake as well as the fruits and vegetables in her diet and the amount of water she drank. At the same time, I slowly increased our workouts. After three months, Margaret was driving herself to the gym rather than having her daughter drive her. She started wearing some makeup and paying more attention to how she dressed—in short, she began to care about herself. After working with me for about a year, she was a different person. She said that she felt twenty years younger, her muscle tone came back, she started feeling hungry again, she was now sleeping six or seven hours a night, and she had started reading again because her concentration had improved so much.

Shortly after that, Margaret moved to a retirement community in Florida, but we've stayed in touch. She tells me that she has continued to work out and to eat healthy meals. Now, five years later, she has a boyfriend who is ten years younger than she is. She has become an organizer in her community and is trying to get her fellow residents to become more active.

To me, Margaret is proof that it's never too old to start getting healthy.

How Long Can We Really Live?

The World Health Organization tells us that life expectancy increased five years between 2000 and 2015 (the last year for which statistics are available).[2] And according to an article by Gregg Easterbrook in the *Atlantic*, life expectancy in America at the beginning of the twentieth century was just forty-seven years, while the life expectancy of a newborn today is seventy-nine years. If we continue at that rate, American life expectancy by the end of the twenty-first century will be one hundred years. These projections do not assume any spectacular medical discoveries, just an ever-longer ride on what the author refers to as a rising escalator. And if science does come up with new antiaging drugs or genetic therapies, living to be one hundred may become the norm rather than the exception.[3]

Furthermore, researchers at the University Research Institute of Gerontology and Metabolism in Madrid, Spain, used a mathematical model of growth and survival rates to study human life span. They concluded, "Human life span seems to be limited up to around 120 years, but growth process modulating factors could theoretically enhance it."[4]

Based on this information, we must all do whatever we can to ensure that we live as long and as well as we possibly can. The Fountain of Youth is actually already within our grasp.

ReSYNC Your Way to a Longer, More Fulfilling Life

I can't promise that you'll live to be 120, or even 100 years old. And I can't promise that you'll never get sick. But I can promise that if you keep exercising and eating well for the rest of your life, you'll live longer, better, smarter, and with a closer relationship to God than if you go back to your old ways of being. But I'm also confident that after twenty-eight days you won't want to regress. I've heard it time and again—people come up to me and say, "Oh, Samir, I never knew I could feel this way. Thank you so much for showing me how much better I could feel. It's almost as if I've been reborn." Well, there's no need to thank me. Just knowing that I've been able to change your life for the better—and that you're continuing to do what I've taught you—is all the thanks I need.

Keep Moving

Of course, I would love for you to do as much exercise as you can at whatever level you're able. I both hope and believe that once you've completed the twenty-eight-day ReSYNC program, you'll feel and look so much better that you'll be as addicted to moving as you once were to potato chips. You'll love the compliments you receive and the feel-good endorphins that flood your brain when you work out. But again, I want you to understand that you don't have to live at the gym to reap the benefits of getting yourself to move.

The most recent Physical Activity Guidelines for Americans recommend 75 minutes of vigorous intensity or 150 minutes of moderate intensity aerobic activity per week, but studies have shown a 20 percent reduction in mortality rate among those who did less than the recommended amount when compared with those who did no exercise at all.[5]

Eat Well

Like exercise, eating good, clean, unprocessed foods for at least the last month will have cleansed your body of a lifetime of unhealthy toxins and changed the way you think about what you eat. It will also have changed the way you digest and metabolize whatever you consume. No, you won't magically have developed the ability to burn off all the calories in a T-bone steak and fries or regularly consume an entire box of doughnuts without any detrimental effects, but you probably won't want to do that anyway, because it's going to make you feel sick. Maybe you used to think that it was normal to feel stuffed and sluggish most of the time, but now you know it's not.

The good news is that once you've reached a healthy weight and you're getting regular exercise, you won't have to think so much about portion size, because you'll know what a healthy portion should be, and you'll also be able to expand your food choices. I don't want to keep you on a weight-loss diet forever—because you wouldn't stick to it—nobody does. What I want to do is give you a road map to follow so that you stay on course for the rest of your life. Here's a list of fifty healthy foods that will help you do that. If you eat these foods regularly, you'll be consuming healthy proteins, complex carbs, and good fats. You'll be getting all the vitamins and minerals you need, along with the antioxidants that fight inflammation. And you'll cut down the damage done by free radicals that could shorten your life.

Fifty Foods to Have on Hand at All Times

1. **Asparagus.** Contains a chemical that helps break down fat and remove it from your body.

2. **Avocados.** Rich and creamy in texture, avocados are packed with monounsaturated fat that can help lower bad (LDL) and raise good (HDL) cholesterol. Enjoy them in salads or as guacamole (which also contains tomatoes and onions, two of the other foods on your must-have list).

3. **Beans and legumes.** Lentils, chickpeas, black beans, fava beans, kidney beans, lima beans, pinto beans, and cannellini beans are a great vegetarian source of protein as well as being high in fiber and low in fat.

4. **Beef (lean).** Lean beef can be incorporated into your healthy diet. Look for the following cuts: eye of round, sirloin tip side steak, top sirloin, bottom round, filet mignon, and skirt steak.

5. **Beets.** Sweet and delicious in salads or as a side dish, beets are rich in vitamin C as well as potassium, manganese, and folate.

6. **Bell peppers (red, green, and yellow).** The color is actually determined by how long the pepper has been allowed to ripen on the vine. While all colors contain significant amounts of nutrients, red bell peppers have the most, including vitamins A and C, potassium, and folic acid, because they have been allowed to ripen the longest.

7. **Celery.** In addition to providing a satisfying crunch with virtually no calories (one medium rib has six calories), celery contains a wide variety of healthy antioxidants, including vitamin C, beta-carotene, and manganese.

8. **Cheese (reduced-fat).** Everyone loves cheese, and it's filled with calcium, which is good for bones and teeth. It also has a lot of protein—great for vegetarians. But it is also calorie dense, so don't overdo, and try to stick with low- or reduced-fat versions of your favorites.

9. **Chili peppers.** Capsaicin, the compound that gives varieties of chilies their heat, also helps break down and eliminate stored body fat.

10. **Citrus fruit.** Oranges, grapefruit, lemons, and limes are all rich in vitamin C and good sources of antioxidants.

11. **Coconut.** It improves the body's ability to absorb calcium and magnesium, which contribute to healthy bones and teeth. The meat contains vitamins A and E along with phytochemicals that work together to decrease levels of LDL (bad) cholesterol and reduce your risk for cardiovascular diseases. Almost 50 percent of the fatty acid in coconut is composed of lauric acid, which has antimicrobial properties that fight against bacteria, viruses, and other pathogens in the body. Grate the meat on salads or eat it out of hand, try coconut milk, or cook with coconut oil.

12. **Coffee.** Yes, coffee! It's a rich source of antioxidants, and according to several recent studies, it may help reduce your risk of type 2 diabetes and Parkinson's disease, as well as various types of cancer.

13. **Cruciferous vegetables.** Broccoli, cauliflower, cabbage, and Brussels sprouts, as well as other cruciferous vegetables, protect against oxidative stress, which helps lower your risk of cardiovascular disease as well as various forms of cancer. To retain their maximum benefits, eat them raw or only lightly cooked.

14. **Cucumbers.** Made up of approximately 95 percent water, cucumbers are hydrating and low in calories, but they also pack a nutritional punch. Cucumbers contain B vitamins as well as vitamins C and K, along with copper, manganese, and potassium. Plus, cucumbers contain unique polyphenols and other compounds that may help reduce your risk of chronic diseases and much, much more.

15. **Dark chocolate (75 percent or more cacao).** Contains high levels

of the antioxidant flavenol. Just one-third ounce will help satisfy your sweet tooth.

16. **Eggplant.** Rich in vitamins and minerals, and the skin contains an antioxidant that aids in cell protection and regeneration. One cup of cubed eggplant contains only twenty calories.

17. **Eggs (cage-free).** A good source of protein. Eating an egg at breakfast will keep you full longer than if you ate only a bagel or toast, for example. Eggs contain choline, which helps with brain development and mental alertness, while the chemicals lutein and zeaxanthin have been associated with protecting you from developing cataracts.

18. **Fish and shellfish.** In addition to being a great source of lean protein, fish is high in omega-3 fatty acids, which help reduce risk factors for heart disease, including high cholesterol and high blood pressure. Look for wild salmon, mackerel, tuna, and sardines. In addition to being low in fat and calories, shrimp is a good source of the antioxidant mineral selenium. Mussels contain extremely high levels of vitamin B_{12}, which helps your brain stay sharp as you age.

19. **Fresh fruits and berries.** Apples, bananas, apricots, guavas, papaya, kiwis, cherries, strawberries, pineapple, blueberries, cranberries, and raspberries, among others, are all high in antioxidants and fiber that protect your health and aid digestion at the same time they provide satisfaction to your sweet tooth.

20. **Garlic (fresh).** No wonder legend tells us that garlic wards off evil spirits. A member of the onion family, it has many health benefits, including a sulfur compound called allicin, which boosts the immune system, has been shown to lower LDL (bad) cholesterol and raise HDL (good) cholesterol, and lower your risk of heart attack and stroke by improving the function of the circulatory system.

21. **Greek yogurt.** Containing about twice as much protein as regular yogurt, Greek yogurt is high in calcium and vitamin B$_{12}$. It is also packed with probiotics that boost your immune system and balance the bacteria in your gut.

22. **Green peas and green beans.** String beans are the most common type of green beans, but there are a number of varieties, all of which have approximately the same health properties. High in fiber and low in calories, they are a great source of vitamins, such as A, C, K, B$_6$, and folic acid, as well as calcium, silicon, iron, manganese, potassium, and copper. When they're young and fresh, enjoy munching on them raw, and if you do cook them, don't overdo it—they should still be bright green and crisp when they're done. Sweet peas are sweet for a reason—they contain sugar, but they also contain phytonutrients with key antioxidant and anti-inflammatory benefits. And although they are extremely low in fat, they are a reliable source of omega-3 and omega-6 fatty acids. For a healthy sweet treat, eat your peas right out of the shell.

23. **Honey.** Use it as a sweetener instead of refined sugar. Unlike sugar, honey has many health benefits. A natural cough suppressant, it also contains tryptophan, which helps relax you so that you are able to get a good night's sleep. Stir it into a cup of tea before you go to bed.

24. **Hummus.** A delicious dip or spread made with chickpeas, olive oil, garlic, lemon juice, and sesame seed paste, hummus contains nothing but healthy ingredients. Spread it on a whole-grain cracker, or use it as a dip for raw vegetables, such as celery, carrot sticks, or bell pepper strips.

25. **Leafy green vegetables.** Spinach, kale, collards, Swiss chard, and dark green lettuces are, calorie for calorie, more nutritious than any other food. They're packed with a wide variety of vitamins and minerals as well as fiber and phytochemicals that fight free radicals and inflammation.

26. **Melons.** Watermelon is not only sweet and juicy, it also contains citrulline, an amino acid that is good for the cardiovascular system. Cantaloupe contains high levels of vitamins A and C as well as potassium and magnesium, among other healthy vitamins and minerals. Honeydew melon is also high in vitamin C and potassium as well as iron and B vitamins. All melons make for a refreshing and hydrating healthy, sweet dessert.

27. **Mushrooms.** Available in many varieties and extremely low in calories, mushrooms contain selenium as well as a particular type of fiber called beta-glucan, which the body cannot manufacture. Both selenium and beta-glucan boost the immune system and help fight infections. Try a healthy, low-cal, meaty-tasting grilled portobello mushroom instead of a burger, or eat mushrooms raw in salads, in sauces, or as a topping.

28. **Nuts and seeds.** Nuts and seeds are high in fiber and contain mono- and polyunsaturated heart-healthy fats. Try flax seeds, pumpkin seeds, sunflower seeds, peanuts (actually a legume), chia seeds, walnuts, raw almonds, macadamia nuts, and Brazil nuts.

29. **Oatmeal (steel cut).** Loaded with fiber, oatmeal helps reduce LDL (bad) cholesterol and can help regulate blood sugar as well as keep you feeling full longer.

30. **Oils.** Olive oil is high in monounsaturated fats and helps lower LDL (bad) cholesterol. Avocado oil and almond oil are also great sources of monounsaturated fat. Flaxseed oil, walnut oil, and hemp oil are all rich in essential omega-3 fatty acids. Coconut oil and its cousin red palm oil both contain high levels of health-promoting antioxidants. Sesame oil, most often used in Asian cooking, is extremely tasty and is rich in the minerals iron, calcium, and magnesium as well as polyunsaturated fat.

31. **Okra.** High in fiber, vitamins, and minerals, okra can help control cholesterol and aid in weight reduction.

32. **Olives.** Yes, they are little balls of fat, but it is healthy, monounsaturated fat, which has been shown to reduce LDL (bad) cholesterol levels and can help lower blood pressure. They also contain an extremely wide variety of antioxidant and anti-inflammatory nutrients. Just don't overdo, because, as I said, whatever their health benefits, they are still tiny balls of fat.

33. **Onions.** From sweet to tangy, onions are full of health benefits. In addition to vitamin C, they contain quercetin, which has been associated with reducing the risk for cancer, and chromium, which helps regulate blood sugar. For centuries onions have been used to reduce inflammation and heal infections, as well as to take the sting out of bee stings.

34. **Orange-colored vegetables.** Carrots, sweet potatoes, and squash are rich in vitamin A and beta-carotene. Eat them cooked to get the most benefit from the powerful phytochemicals they contain.

35. **Peanut butter and almond butter (preferably all-natural).** Although they're high in fat, peanut and almond butter also contain protein (8 grams in two tablespoons for peanut butter; almost 7 grams for almond butter), so spreading some on your morning whole-grain toast will keep you feeling fuller longer.

36. **Pomegranates.** Sweet-tart and delicious, pomegranates, including their seeds and juice, pack a tremendous antioxidant punch.

37. **Popcorn.** That's right: your favorite movie snack is actually good for your health. Popcorn is a whole grain that provides fiber and antioxidants. Just stay away from the butter!

38. **Pork.** Look for tenderloin, rib chops, sirloin roast, or top-loin chops.

39. **Poultry.** White meat chicken is leaner than dark meat, and most of the fat is in the skin. If you remove the skin before cooking, you'll prevent the fat from melting into the meat. Therefore skinless, boneless

chicken breast is the leanest of the lean. While a three-ounce portion of skinless turkey breast provides the same amount of protein as a three-ounce portion of skinless chicken breast, the turkey is slightly lower in calories. Interestingly, however, dark meat turkey is slightly higher in calories than dark meat chicken. And if you're thinking of switching from beef to turkey burgers, make sure that the ground turkey you buy is all-white meat, with no skin included—otherwise you might be better off with extra-lean ground beef.

40. **Prunes.** A tasty sweet treat and a good source of energy that doesn't spike blood sugar, probably because they're high in fiber. Just be careful not to overdo—not only are prunes relatively high in calories, but the sorbitol they contain acts as a laxative.

41. **Quinoa.** A grain that deserves a category all its own, quinoa not only is rich in a variety of antioxidants with more heart-healthy monounsaturated fats than plant foods, but it also is the only plant source of complete protein, meaning that it contains all the essential fatty acids our bodies cannot manufacture for themselves.

42. **Rice (brown, black, or wild).** Unlike white rice, both brown rice and black rice retain the hull and the bran, which makes them whole grains. Brown and black rice are rich in protein, thiamine, calcium, magnesium, and potassium, and because they have so much fiber, they do not cause a spike in blood sugar levels. Black rice is even lower in calories and higher in fiber; it's also a better source of protein than brown rice. Wild rice is actually a grass that produces a grain and is only distantly related to other types of rice. It is exceptionally nutritious, containing high amounts of vitamins and minerals as well as protein.

43. **Salsa.** There's a good reason why salsa has become so popular. Usually made with tomatoes and fresh vegetables with hot chilies added, it has all the health benefits of each of its individual ingredients.

44. **Soy and tofu.** Low in saturated fat, soy is a good source of lean, heart-healthy protein. Try edamame (fresh soybeans). Tofu is made from coagulated soy milk that is compressed and cut into squares. Soy milk is also a great alternative to cow's milk for people who are lactose intolerant.

45. **Spices.** Ginger, cayenne, cinnamon, and turmeric, for example, add flavor without adding calories and contain anti-inflammatory agents. Keep a variety of spices in your pantry to flavor your favorite dishes.

46. **Tea.** Green tea contains antioxidants and nutrients that, among other health benefits, improve brain function, help increase weight loss, and lower the risk for cancer. Chamomile tea soothes anxiety and is a natural sleep aid.

47. **Tomatoes.** Tomatoes are probably best known as the richest source of lycopene, a carotenoid that gives them their rich, red color and also helps destroy free radicals and protect against a variety of cancers. While in most cases fruits and vegetables are most nutritious in their raw state, the lycopene is more bioavailable when the tomatoes are cooked—as in sauce, ketchup, tomato paste, or tomato soup.

48. **Vinegar.** The acetic acid in vinegar helps stabilize blood sugar levels after eating.

49. **Wheat bran cereal.** Be sure that you're buying high-fiber, 100 percent bran cereal, without added sugar. It's been shown to help improve your mood and your mind, and it provides great energy.

50. **Whole-grain bread.** First of all, make sure that the bread you buy is "100 percent" whole grain. Some breads will say they "contain" whole wheat or whole grains, but that's not the same thing. Whole grains are packed with nutrients, including protein, fiber, B vitamins, antioxidants, and trace amounts of iron, zinc, copper, and magnesium. Diets rich in whole grains have been shown to reduce the risk of heart disease, type 2 diabetes, obesity, and some forms of cancer.

Don't Be Too Hard on Yourself

Indulge yourself once in a while (and that "once in a while" is the key), so long as you don't then feel guilty about it or decide that you've "blown it anyway" so you might as well just give up. Is it your birthday? By all means have a piece of cake. Thanksgiving? How about a small piece of pumpkin pie? The thing is, I don't want you to think that you can never have a dessert again for the rest of your life. That just isn't realistic.

My goal is for you to be healthy and happy—not skinny and miserable.

Sleep!

One area I haven't yet mentioned but that is significant for success in every aspect of your life is sleep. Aside from drinking more water, if I could get you to change just one habit for the better, it would be to get enough (but not too much) sleep. Although I almost never hear anyone say they're sleeping too much (unless it's associated with some other condition, such as depression), almost everyone complains about not getting enough sleep. Whether it's because there aren't enough hours in the day to get everything done (or so they think) or they simply can't get to sleep because they're too stressed or thinking too much, people just don't seem to be able to get a good night's rest. And that's a serious problem!

Clint, one of my clients, was a small business owner who constantly complained that he could never get to sleep because he couldn't "turn off his brain." He was always thinking about his business, what he needed to get done, and how he was going to expand it even more. Married, with a son and a daughter, he was forty-five at the time, six feet three inches tall, and 230 pounds. He was a real family man and a regular churchgoer. His wife, a stay-at-home mom, cooked healthy meals, and the family as a whole led a pretty healthy lifestyle. Clint had no problem getting started on the ReSYNC program, but I found that whenever we met, all he wanted to talk about was his business. After about a week, I told him I was making a new rule: no talking about business when he was with me. He could pick any other topic he wanted, but we would not discuss his work. I also suggested that in addition to going to church, he should take a few quiet moments each day to pray or meditate. The problem for Clint was that he had totally lost contact with his body and with who he was (other than the owner of his business).

To help him get to sleep, I told him not to eat any heavy carbs in the evening and to turn off all his electronics at least half an hour before he went to bed.

Clint lost thirty pounds on the program, but that wasn't the most important change for him. The important thing was that he finally was able to get a good night's rest. And his wife was happy to report that when he came home in the evening, he was no longer talking about work. Clint realized that once he was sleeping better, he had more energy and was more focused when he got up in the morning. As a result, he was working more efficiently and no longer had to spend his evenings thinking about and catching up on the work he hadn't done during the day.

In addition to affecting mental alertness, getting a good night's sleep is crucial for losing weight, for building muscle, and for maintaining a healthy digestive system. Sleep deprivation can lead to serious medical conditions, including diabetes, high blood pressure, and stroke.[6]

Lack of sleep has been linked to an increased level of C-reactive protein, which is associated with a higher risk of death from cardiovascular disease.[7] And studies have shown that people who don't get enough sleep are heavier than those who do.[8] Lack of sleep seems to affect weight in a number of ways: people who are tired tend not to exercise, people who are awake longer tend to eat more, and lack of sleep disrupts the balance of hormones that affect appetite.[9] For example, studies have shown that only six days of sleep deprivation can lead to a decrease in the hormone leptin, which signals satiety, and just two days of sleep restriction results in increased levels of ghrelin, which stimulates appetite. The conclusion is that loss of sleep "seems to alter the ability of leptin and ghrelin to accurately signal caloric need and could lead to excessive caloric intake when food is freely available." The findings also suggest that "compliance with a weight-loss diet involving caloric restriction may be adversely affected by sleep restriction."[10]

But *when* you go to sleep is as important as *how much* sleep you get. You need to get to sleep before midnight because the ratio of deep (non-REM) sleep to lighter (REM) sleep decreases as the night wears on, and it's important to get as much deep sleep as you can. I recommend that you go to sleep by ten o'clock and not eat anything or drink too much water within ninety minutes of when you go to bed. Your digestive system needs rest too. And, of course, if you drink too much too close to bedtime, you'll be getting up in the middle of the night and disturbing your rest to go to the bathroom.

Here are a few more tips for getting a better night's sleep:

- Make sure the room is as dark as possible.
- Make sure the room is cool—no more than 70 degrees.
- Reserve your bed for sleeping only—no doing work or watching television.
- Go to bed at the same time every night, including weekends.
- Take some time to wind down; don't engage in stimulating activities right before bedtime.[11]

Keep Drinking Water

Without repeating all the reasons we discussed in chapter 3, I must remind you how important it is to drink water before meals, after having coffee or tea, and regularly throughout the day to remain hydrated and keep your body functioning at its peak.

Take Care of Your Oral Health

Many people don't realize that the bacteria we all have in our mouths can affect the health of the rest of our body. Oral bacteria have been linked to endocarditis, an inflammation of the inner lining of the heart, as well as to cardiovascular disease. So, please, take good care of your teeth and gums.

Stay Connected

Maintaining social connections as well as the support of your family is as important for longevity as maintaining a healthy lifestyle.

In chapter 5 we discussed the fact that belonging to a spiritual community provides a support system that helps reduce stress and protect us from disease. I've always been impressed and moved by the way the members of the church community support one another's efforts. If people see that someone is struggling, they often give that person a hug and a few words of encouragement.

Now, researchers at the University of North Carolina at Chapel Hill report that having supportive social relationships is associated with a reduction in the risk for specific conditions that lower life expectancy, including abdominal fat, inflammation, and high blood pressure.[12] And another study, done at Brigham Young University, found that social isolation is as much a risk factor for mortality as obesity.[13]

Nurture Your Spirituality

More than one study has shown that people who attend religious services at least once a week are less likely to die in a given follow-up period than those who don't.[14]

While I personally am not in a position to quantify how much longer regular churchgoers may live than those who don't attend church, I do know that in addition to having a strong support group and a close relationship with God, those people who do attend church services regularly are also less likely to engage in certain life-threatening habits, such as smoking and excessive drinking. And it appears that research backs up my personal observations.[15]

Clearly, there are many reasons to nurture your spirituality, but the possibility of living longer is certainly one of them!

And of Course . . .

It should go without saying that you need to wash your hands frequently to get rid of germs; if you smoke, you really need to quit; and if you drink alcohol, you should do so wisely and in moderation.

My final wish for you: Live long. Be happy and healthy, and prosper.

The ReSYNC Exercise Plan

Individual Exercises

Level 1:1 (10 Minutes)

Warm-Up: Power Walk (1 minute).

Exercise 1: Tension Walk (1 minute).

Active Rest: Shrug Walk (1 minute).

Exercise 2: Hercules Push (30 seconds on each leg).

Active Rest: Frankenstein Walk (1 minute).

Exercise 3: Achilles Tension Squat (Do at least 20 reps in 1 minute).

Active Rest: Penguin Walk (1 minute).

Exercise 4: Ares Side Push (30 seconds on each side).

Active Rest: Superman Walk (1 minute).

Exercise 5: Sisyphus Push (30 seconds on each side).

Level 1:2 (25 minutes)

Warm-Up: Power Walk (1 minute).

Exercise 1: Tension Walk (1 minute).

Active Rest: Shrug Walk (1 minute).

Exercise 2: Hercules Push (30 seconds on each leg).

Active Rest: Frankenstein Walk (1 minute).

Exercise 3: Achilles Tension Squat (Do at least 20 reps in 1 minute).

Active Rest: Penguin Walk (1 minute).

Exercise 4: Ares Side Push (30 seconds on each side).

Active Rest: Superman Walk (1 minute).

Exercise 5: Sisyphus Push (30 seconds on each side).

Take a 5-minute rest.

Warm-Up: Power Walk (1 minute).

Exercise 1: Tension Walk (1 minute).

Active Rest: Shrug Walk (1 minute).

Exercise 2: Hercules Push (30 seconds on each leg).

Active Rest: Frankenstein Walk (1 minute).

Exercise 3: Achilles Tension Squat (Do at least 20 reps in 1 minute).

Active Rest: Penguin Walk (1 minute).

Exercise 4: Ares Side Push (30 seconds on each side).

Active Rest: Superman Walk (1 minute).

Exercise 5: Sisyphus Push (30 seconds on each side).

Level 2:1 (25 Minutes)

Warm Up: Power Run (1 minute).

Exercise 1: Push-Up-and-a-Half (1 minute).

Active Rest: Shrug Run (1 minute).

Exercise 2: Aphrodite Squat (1 minute).

Active Rest: Frankenstein Run (1 minute).

Exercise 3: Pharaoh Dance (1 minute).

Active Rest: Penguin Run (1 minute).

Exercise 4: Samson Pose (30 seconds on each side).

Active Rest: Superman Run (1 minute).

Exercise 5: Atlas Pose (30 seconds on each side).

Take a 5-minute rest.

Exercise 6: Tension Run (1 minute).

Active Rest: Shrug Run (1 minute).

Exercise 7: Hercules Push (30 seconds on each leg).

Active Rest: Frankenstein Run (1 minute).

Exercise 8: Achilles Tension Squat (Do at least 20 reps in 1 minute).

Active Rest: Penguin Run (1 minute).

Exercise 9: Ares Side Push (30 seconds on each side).

Active Rest: Superman Run (1 minute).

Exercise 10: Sisyphus Push (30 seconds on each side).

Level 2:2 (45 Minutes)

Warm Up: Power Run (1 minute).

Exercise 1: Push-Up-and-a-Half (1 minute).

Active Rest: Shrug Run (1 minute).

Exercise 2: Aphrodite Squat (1 minute).

Active Rest: Frankenstein Run (1 minute).

Exercise 3: Pharaoh Dance (1 minute).

Active Rest: Penguin Run (1 minute).

Exercise 4: Samson Pose (30 seconds on each side).

Active Rest: Superman Run (1 minute).

Exercise 5: Atlas Pose (30 seconds on each side).

Exercise 6: Tension Run (1 minute).

Active Rest: Shrug Run (1 minute).

Exercise 7: Hercules Push (30 seconds on each leg).

Active Rest: Frankenstein Run (1 minute).

Exercise 8: Achilles Tension Squat (Do at least 20 reps in 1 minute).

Active Rest: Penguin Run (1 minute).

Exercise 9: Ares Side Push (30 seconds on each side).

Active Rest: Superman Run (1 minute).

Exercise 10: Sisyphus Push (30 seconds on each side).

Take a 5-minute rest.

Warm Up: Power Run (1 minute).

Exercise 1: Push-Up-and-a-Half (1 minute).

Active Rest: Shrug Run (1 minute).

Exercise 2: Aphrodite Squat (1 minute).

Active Rest: Frankenstein Run (1 minute).

Exercise 3: Pharaoh Dance (1 minute).

Active Rest: Penguin Run (1 minute).

Exercise 4: Samson Pose (30 seconds on each side).

Active Rest: Superman Run (1 minute).

Exercise 5: Atlas Pose (30 seconds on each side).

Exercise 6: Tension Run (1 minute).

Active Rest: Shrug Run (1 minute).

Exercise 7: Hercules Push (30 seconds on each leg).

Active Rest: Frankenstein Run (1 minute).

Exercise 8: Achilles Tension Squat (Do at least 20 reps in 1 minute).

Active Rest: Penguin Run (1 minute).

Exercise 9: Ares Side Push (30 seconds on each side).

Active Rest: Superman Run (1 minute).

Exercise 10: Sisyphus Push (30 seconds on each side).

Partner Exercises

Level 1:1 (10 Minutes)

Warm Up: Power Walk (1 minute).

Partner Exercise 1: Compromise (1 minute).

Active Rest: Shrug Walk (1 Minute).

Partner Exercise 2: Synchronize (1 minute).

Active Rest: Frankenstein Walk (1 minute).

Partner Exercise 3: Support (1 minute).

Active Rest: Penguin Walk (1 minute).

Partner Exercise 4: Trust (1 minute).

Active Rest: Superman Walk (1 minute).

Partner Exercise 5: Harmony (1 minute).

Level 2:1 (25 Minutes)

Warm Up: Power Walk (1 minute).

Partner Exercise 1: Compromise (1 minute).

Active Rest: Shrug Walk (1 Minute).

Partner Exercise 2: Synchronize (1 minute).

Active Rest: Frankenstein Walk (1 minute).

Partner Exercise 3: Support (1 minute).

Active Rest: Penguin Walk (1 minute).

Partner Exercise 4: Trust (1 minute).

Active Rest: Superman Walk (1 minute).

Partner Exercise 5: Harmony (1 minute).

Take a 5-minute rest.

Warm Up: Power Walk (1 minute).

Partner Exercise 1: Compromise (1 minute).

Active Rest: Shrug Walk (1 Minute).

Partner Exercise 2: Synchronize (1 minute).

Active Rest: Frankenstein Walk (1 minute).

Partner Exercise 3: Support (1 minute).

Active Rest: Penguin Walk (1 minute).

Partner Exercise 4: Trust (1 minute).

Active Rest: Superman Walk (1 minute).

Partner Exercise 5: Harmony (1 minute).

Level 2:1 (20 Minutes)

Warm Up: Power Walk (1 minute).

Partner Exercise 1: Compromise (2 minutes).

Active Rest: Shrug Walk (2 Minutes).

Partner Exercise 2: Synchronize (2 minutes).

Active Rest: Frankenstein Walk (2 minutes).

Partner Exercise 3: Support (2 minutes).

Active Rest: Penguin Walk (2 minutes).

Partner Exercise 4: Trust (2 minutes).

Active Rest: Superman Walk (2 minutes).

Partner Exercise 5: Harmony (2 minutes).

Level 2:2 (45 Minutes)

Warm Up: Power Walk (1 minute).

Partner Exercise 1: Compromise (2 minutes).

Active Rest: Shrug Walk (2 Minutes).

Partner Exercise 2: Synchronize (2 minutes).

Active Rest: Frankenstein Walk (2 minutes).

Partner Exercise 3: Support (2 minutes).

Active Rest: Penguin Walk (2 minutes).

Partner Exercise 4: Trust (2 minutes).

Active Rest: Superman Walk (2 minutes).

Partner Exercise 5: Harmony (2 minutes).

Take a 5-minute rest.

Warm Up: Power Walk (1 minute).

Partner Exercise 1: Compromise (2 minutes).

Active Rest: Shrug Walk (2 Minutes).

Partner Exercise 2: Synchronize (2 minutes).

Active Rest: Frankenstein Walk (2 minutes).

Partner Exercise 3: Support (2 minutes).

Active Rest: Penguin Walk (2 minutes).

Partner Exercise 4: Trust (2 minutes).

Active Rest: Superman Walk (2 minutes).

Partner Exercise 5: Harmony (2 minutes).

Seated Exercises

Exercise 1: Upper-Body Tense (Hold for 30 seconds; repeat 4 times).

Exercise 2: Tension Shoulder Press (Repeat 10 times; do 4 sets total).

Exercise 3: Tension Chest Press-Pull (Do 4 sets with a 30-second break between each set).

Exercise 4: Leg Tension (Hold for 30 seconds, repeat 4 times).

Exercise 5: Full Body Tension (4 sets with a 30-second break between each).

Recipe List

Dressings

Basil Pesto

Combine 1 cup fresh basil, 2 tablespoons pine nuts, $\frac{1}{2}$ avocado, 1 garlic clove, juice of $\frac{1}{2}$ lemon, and 3 tablespoons water in food processor and pulse for 20 seconds.

Cilantro Yogurt Dressing

Combine 1 cup chopped cilantro, $\frac{1}{2}$ cup Greek yogurt, 1 pressed garlic clove, 2 teaspoons olive oil, juice of 1 lemon, and salt and pepper to taste. Mix well.

Dijon Mustard Dressing

Combine 1 teaspoon olive oil, $\frac{1}{2}$ teaspoon Dijon mustard, 1 teaspoon organic apple cider vinegar, and salt and pepper to taste. Mix well.

Week One

Breakfast Options

1. **Berry Yogurt.** Greek yogurt mixed with berries and flax seeds

2. **Veggie Eggs.** Two eggs, 1/2 slice of Mestemacher Fitness Bread, and a side of tomatoes and cucumbers

3. **Breakfast Smoothie.** Blend 1 cup Greek yogurt, 1 cup frozen berries, 1 teaspoon flaxseed, and 1 cup ice.

Lunch Options

1. **Chicken and Veggies.** 6 ounces poached boneless, skinless chicken breast, chopped or shredded, combined with 1 cup cherry tomatoes, 1 teaspoon chopped sun-dried tomato, and 1/2 cup raw or blanched chopped asparagus spears. Season with salt, pepper, and fresh basil.

2. **Chicken and Vegetable Soup.** Soup made with reduced-sodium chicken broth, chopped cooked chicken breast, and chopped vegetables from the week one carb options. Serve with leafy greens of your choice sautéed in 1 tablespoon olive oil and seasoned with cayenne pepper.

3. **Snapper and Veggies.** 4 ounces grilled snapper fillet served with grilled mixed vegetables from the week one carb options.

Dinner Options

1. **Lemon Chicken.** 6 ounces grilled boneless, skinless chicken breast served with grilled vegetables from the week one carb options, sprinkled with finely grated lemon zest and chopped fresh thyme.

2. **Grilled Halibut.** 4 ounces grilled halibut, seasoned with cayenne pepper and served with steamed broccoli and a side salad dressed with 1 tablespoon of olive oil and balsamic vinegar.

3. **Grilled Fish Tacos.** 4 ounces of fish of your choice, diced tomato, green peppers, and onions, seasoned with cayenne pepper and wrapped in lettuce leaves.

Week Two

Breakfast Options

1. **Poached Eggs.** Two poached eggs with grilled or steamed asparagus.

2. **Egg White Omelet.** Combine 4 egg whites, chopped bell pepper, celery, onions, and tomatoes, and serve with ½ slice Mestamacher Fitness Bread.

3. **Veggie Quiche Cup.** Chop a mix of your favorite veggies and place in muffin cup, filling it halfway. In bowl, whisk 2 eggs with salt and pepper (add herbs of your choice if desired), and pour over veggies, filling muffin cup to within ¼ inch of top. Bake for 20 to 25 minutes at 350 degrees. Scoop onto plate and enjoy.

Lunch Options

1. **Tomato Soup Smoothie.** In blender, combine 2 large, ripe, peeled tomatoes, 1 cup plain Greek yogurt, and a pinch of fresh basil. Blend until smooth and season with salt and pepper.

2. **Chicken and Cabbage.** Combine 2 cups shredded cabbage with 1 cup shredded carrots. Toss with 1 teaspoon olive oil, lemon juice to taste,

and 2 tablespoons chopped fresh dill. Top with 4 ounces grilled skinless, boneless chicken breast.

3. **Roasted Cauliflower.** Toss florets from 1/4-head cauliflower with 1 teaspoon olive oil, 1 chopped garlic clove, salt, and pepper, and roast for 20 minutes at 450 degrees. Serve with 4 ounces grilled shrimp and 2 teaspoons Cilantro Yogurt Dressing (page 88).

Dinner Options

1. **Tuna with Green Beans and Almonds.** Heat 1 tablespoon olive oil in skillet over medium-high heat. Season 4-ounce tuna fillet with salt and pepper, and roll it in sesame seeds. Add fish to pan and cook for 2 to 3 minutes on each side. In second pan, heat 1 tablespoon olive oil. When hot, add 1 chopped garlic clove, a large handful of green beans, and 1/4 cup sliced almonds. Season with sea salt and cook, stirring occasionally, until beans are crisp-tender, for 3 to 5 minutes. Serve beans with tuna.

2. **Grilled Chicken Breast with Brussels Sprouts.** Heat 1 tablespoon olive oil in skillet over medium-high heat. Add chopped Brussels sprouts and cook, stirring, until softened. Add 1 teaspoon chopped walnuts and season with Dijon Mustard Dressing (page 89). Serve with 4 ounces grilled skinless, boneless chicken breast.

3. **Grilled Portobello Mushrooms with Tomatoes and Eggplant.** Season two Portobello mushrooms with sea salt and olive oil and grill over medium-high heat for 10 minutes. Heat 1 tablespoon olive oil in skillet. When hot, add 1 cup chopped onion and 2 chopped garlic cloves. Cook, stirring until onion is golden brown. Add 2 cups chopped tomato and 1 cup chopped eggplant, and cook, stirring, for another 5 to 10 minutes. To serve, top mushrooms with onion and tomato mixture.

Week Three

Breakfast Options

1. **Overnight Oatmeal.** In container with tight-fitting lid, combine $1/2$ cup raw oats, $1/2$ cup nonfat milk or almond milk, and 1 teaspoon honey. Shake to mix well and refrigerate overnight. In the morning, when ready to eat, add 1 cup fresh berries and 1 teaspoon chopped mixed nuts.

2. **Banana-Chia Smoothie.** In a container with a tight-fitting lid, combine $1/4$ cup chia seeds with $1/2$ cup almond milk and $1/2$ cup coconut milk. Shake to mix well and refrigerate overnight. In the morning, when ready to eat, add $1/2$ chopped banana and 1 teaspoon sliced almonds.

3. **Fruit and Cottage Cheese.** Combine 1 cup cottage cheese with $1/3$ cup chopped plums and 1 tablespoon chopped walnuts.

Lunch Options

1. **Turkey and Lettuce Bowl.** In skillet over medium heat, sauté $1/2$ chopped yellow onion in 1 teaspoon olive oil until soft but not brown. Add 3 ounces ground lean turkey and cook, stirring, until meat is no longer pink. Season with salt and cayenne pepper, and serve in bowl over shredded lettuce, chopped tomatoes, and peppers.

2. **Fish and Sweet Potatoes.** 4 ounces grilled cod fillet served with $1/2$ cup sweet potato purée.

3. **Broccoli and Kale Soup.** Heat 1 tablespoon olive oil in large skillet over medium-high heat. Add 1 chopped garlic clove, 1 teaspoon chopped fresh ginger, $1/2$ teaspoon turmeric, salt and pepper to taste, and cook, stirring, 1 to 2 minutes. Add 2 cups low-sodium vegetable broth and cook 5 minutes

more. Add 1 cup broccoli florets and 2 to 3 cups chopped kale, and cook until broccoli is crisp-tender, 4 to 5 more minutes. Serve in soup bowl, and season with chopped cilantro and lime juice.

Dinner Options

1. **Quinoa and Scallops.** Combine ¹/₂ cup cooked quinoa with ¹/₄ cup chickpeas, ¹/₂ cucumber, cut into cubes, and ¹/₄ head cabbage, shredded. Season with lemon juice and dill (or another herb of your choice), and serve with 3¹/₂ ounces grilled scallops.

2. **Spaghetti Squash with Tomatoes.** Preheat oven to 400 degrees. Cut a spaghetti squash in half and remove seeds. Roast squash for 25 to 40 minutes, until flesh is tender and skin is easily pierced with fork. Use fork to scrape out squash so that it forms spaghetti-like strands. Heat 1 tablespoon olive oil in skillet over medium-high heat. When hot, add ¹/₂ cup cherry tomato halves and cook, stirring, for 3 to 5 minutes. Season with salt and pepper. Add 1 chopped garlic clove and spaghetti squash. Cook, stirring, for 2 minutes longer. Remove from heat and stir in ¹/₂ cup cubed fresh mozzarella cheese. Garnish with snipped fresh basil. Serve with 4 ounces grilled shrimp.

3. **Chicken and Broccoli.** 4 ounces grilled skinless, boneless chicken breast served with grilled or steamed broccoli florets and carrots seasoned with salt and pepper.

Week Four

Breakfast Options

1. **Rice and Egg Bowl.** Place ¹/₂ cup cooked brown rice in bowl. Top with two poached eggs and ¹/₂ avocado, sliced. Season with salt, pepper, and minced green onions.

2. **Banana-Berry Smoothie.** In blender, combine 1 banana, 1 cup almond milk, 1 cup fresh or frozen berries, 1 tablespoon flaxseeds, and 1 cup ice. Blend for 60 seconds.

3. **Egg and Vegetable Stovetop Frittata.** Steam 1 cup chopped mixed vegetables (whatever is fresh and available) for 2 to 3 minutes. In bowl, beat 2 eggs with salt and pepper. Heat nonstick skillet over medium heat. Add vegetables and pour eggs on top. Cover skillet and cook for another 2 minutes (until eggs are done to your taste). Serve with a slice of whole-grain bread.

Lunch Options

1. **Steak and Cukes.** 4 ounces grilled top sirloin or sirloin tip steak served with a side of thinly sliced cucumber, sprinkled with 1 tablespoon sesame seeds and dressed with apple cider vinegar, olive oil, salt, and pepper.

2. **Quinoa Fruit Bowl.** Combine 1/2 cup cooked red quinoa with 1 sliced pear, 2 1/2 ounces fresh baby spinach, and 1/4 cup dried cranberries. Season with lemon juice, salt, and pepper. Serve with 4 ounces grilled chicken.

3. **Pasta and Tomatoes.** Heat 1 tablespoon olive oil in skillet over medium heat. Add 1/2 cup cooked buckwheat pasta, 5 or 6 cherry tomatoes, and 1 teaspoon chopped olives. Cook, stirring, for about 3 minutes. Season with salt, pepper, and fresh basil. Serve with 4 ounces grilled shrimp.

Dinner Options

1. **Scallops and Vegetables.** Heat 1 tablespoon olive oil in skillet over medium-high heat. Add 1/2 cup chopped onion and cook, stirring, until golden brown. Add 1 cup diced sweet potato and cook 15 to 20 minutes. Add 4 ounces scallops and cook 4 to 5 minutes, turning to brown both

sides. When done, remove from the heat and add 2 cups chopped kale. Stir to combine.

2. **Burger Salad.** 4-ounce burger made with ground top or bottom round steak, served over a mixed green salad, dressed with olive oil and apple cider vinegar.

3. **Pesto Pork Chop.** Marinate a 4-ounce rib or loin pork chop in Basil Pesto (page 88) for 30 minutes; then grill over medium-high heat for 5 to 6 minutes on each side. Serve with grilled vegetables of your choice.

The 28-Day ReSYNC
Method Journal

The 28-Day ReSYNC Method Journal

Day 1

Meals

Breakfast	
Snack	
Lunch	
Snack	
Dinner	

The 28-Day ReSYNC Method Journal

Day 1

Workout

Spiritual Practice

Brain Booster

The 28-Day ReSYNC Method Journal

Day 2

Meals

Breakfast	
Snack	
Lunch	
Snack	
Dinner	

The 28-Day ReSYNC Method Journal

Day 2

Workout

Spiritual Practice

Brain Booster

The 28-Day ReSYNC Method Journal

Day 3

Meals

Breakfast	
Snack	
Lunch	
Snack	
Dinner	

The 28-Day ReSYNC Method Journal

Day 3

Workout

Spiritual Practice

Brain Booster

The 28-Day ReSYNC Method Journal

Day 4

Meals

Breakfast	
Snack	
Lunch	
Snack	
Dinner	

The 28-Day ReSYNC Method Journal

Day 4

Workout

Spiritual Practice

Brain Booster

The 28-Day ReSYNC Method Journal

Day 5

Meals

Breakfast	
Snack	
Lunch	
Snack	
Dinner	

The 28-Day ReSYNC Method Journal

Day 5

Workout

Spiritual Practice

Brain Booster

The 28-Day ReSYNC Method Journal

Day 6

Meals

Breakfast	
Snack	
Lunch	
Snack	
Dinner	

The 28-Day ReSYNC Method Journal

Day 6

Workout

Spiritual Practice

Brain Booster

The 28-Day ReSYNC Method Journal

Day 7

Meals

Breakfast	
Snack	
Lunch	
Snack	
Dinner	

The 28-Day ReSYNC Method Journal

Day 7

Workout

Spiritual Practice

Brain Booster

The 28-Day ReSYNC Method Journal

Day 8

Meals

Breakfast	
Snack	
Lunch	
Snack	
Dinner	

The 28-Day ReSYNC Method Journal

Day 8

Workout

Spiritual Practice

Brain Booster

The 28-Day ReSYNC Method Journal

Day 9

Meals

Breakfast	
Snack	
Lunch	
Snack	
Dinner	

The 28-Day ReSYNC Method Journal

Day 9

Workout

Spiritual Practice

Brain Booster

The 28-Day ReSYNC Method Journal

Day 10

Meals

Breakfast	
Snack	
Lunch	
Snack	
Dinner	

The 28-Day ReSYNC Method Journal

Day 10

Workout

Spiritual Practice

Brain Booster

The 28-Day ReSYNC Method Journal

Day 11

Meals

Breakfast	
Snack	
Lunch	
Snack	
Dinner	

The 28-Day ReSYNC Method Journal

Day 11

Workout

Spiritual Practice

Brain Booster

The 28-Day ReSYNC Method Journal

Day 12

Meals

Breakfast	
Snack	
Lunch	
Snack	
Dinner	

The 28-Day ReSYNC Method Journal

Day 12

Workout

Spiritual Practice

Brain Booster

The 28-Day ReSYNC Method Journal

Day 13

Meals

Breakfast	
Snack	
Lunch	
Snack	
Dinner	

The 28-Day ReSYNC Method Journal

Day 13

Workout

Spiritual Practice

Brain Booster

The 28-Day ReSYNC Method Journal

Day 14

Meals

Breakfast	
Snack	
Lunch	
Snack	
Dinner	

The 28-Day ReSYNC Method Journal

Day 14

Workout

Spiritual Practice

Brain Booster

The 28-Day ReSYNC Method Journal

Day 15

Meals

Breakfast	
Snack	
Lunch	
Snack	
Dinner	

The 28-Day ReSYNC Method Journal

Day 15

Workout

Spiritual Practice

Brain Booster

The 28-Day ReSYNC Method Journal

Day 16

Meals

Breakfast	
Snack	
Lunch	
Snack	
Dinner	

The 28-Day ReSYNC Method Journal

Day 16

Workout

Spiritual Practice

Brain Booster

The 28-Day ReSYNC Method Journal

Day 17

Meals

Breakfast	
Snack	
Lunch	
Snack	
Dinner	

The 28-Day ReSYNC Method Journal

Day 17

Workout

Spiritual Practice

Brain Booster

The 28-Day ReSYNC Method Journal

Day 18

Meals

Breakfast	
Snack	
Lunch	
Snack	
Dinner	

The 28-Day ReSYNC Method Journal

Day 18

Workout

Spiritual Practice

Brain Booster

The 28-Day ReSYNC Method Journal

Day 19

Meals

Breakfast	
Snack	
Lunch	
Snack	
Dinner	

The 28-Day ReSYNC Method Journal

Day 19

Workout

Spiritual Practice

Brain Booster

The 28-Day ReSYNC Method Journal

Day 20

Meals

Breakfast	
Snack	
Lunch	
Snack	
Dinner	

The 28-Day ReSYNC Method Journal

Day 20

Workout

Spiritual Practice

Brain Booster

The 28-Day ReSYNC Method Journal

Day 21

Meals

Breakfast	
Snack	
Lunch	
Snack	
Dinner	

The 28-Day ReSYNC Method Journal

Day 21

Workout

Spiritual Practice

Brain Booster

The 28-Day ReSYNC Method Journal

Day 22

Meals

Breakfast	
Snack	
Lunch	
Snack	
Dinner	

The 28-Day ReSYNC Method Journal

Day 22

Workout

Spiritual Practice

Brain Booster

The 28-Day ReSYNC Method Journal

Day 23

Meals

Breakfast	
Snack	
Lunch	
Snack	
Dinner	

The 28-Day ReSYNC Method Journal

Day 23

Workout

Spiritual Practice

Brain Booster

The 28-Day ReSYNC Method Journal

Day 24

Meals

Breakfast	
Snack	
Lunch	
Snack	
Dinner	

The 28-Day ReSYNC Method Journal

Day 24

Workout

Spiritual Practice

Brain Booster

The 28-Day ReSYNC Method Journal

Day 25

Meals

Breakfast	
Snack	
Lunch	
Snack	
Dinner	

The 28-Day ReSYNC Method Journal

Day 25

Workout

Spiritual Practice

Brain Booster

The 28-Day ReSYNC Method Journal

Day 26

Meals

Breakfast	
Snack	
Lunch	
Snack	
Dinner	

The 28-Day ReSYNC Method Journal

Day 26

Workout

Spiritual Practice

Brain Booster

The 28-Day ReSYNC Method Journal

Day 27

Meals

Breakfast	
Snack	
Lunch	
Snack	
Dinner	

The 28-Day ReSYNC Method Journal

Day 27

Workout

Spiritual Practice

Brain Booster

The 28-Day ReSYNC Method Journal

Day 28

Meals

Breakfast	
Snack	
Lunch	
Snack	
Dinner	

The 28-Day ReSYNC Method Journal

Day 28

Workout

Spiritual Practice

Brain Booster

Acknowledgments

I would like to express my deepest gratitude to Eileen Cope, my warrior agent, for her never-ending support and protection. Judy Kern, for putting up with me. Eve Minkler, for inspiring me.

Thank you to the HarperCollins/Thomas Nelson team for being professional, supportive, and just incredible. Brian Hampton, for believing in me. Jenny Baumgartner, for your kindness and work ethic. Brigitta Nortker, Aryn VanDyke, Sara Broun, and Belinda Bass, for your constant support.

To my Health Fitness Revolution team, thank you for being crusaders against obesity. Robert Madden, for being a true friend. My assistant Naomi Ring, for always being on my side. My wife, Dijana, and son, Ares Max, for your never-ending love and devotion.

About the Author

Samir Becic has become an internationally recognized fitness expert, named four times the number one trainer in the United States by Bally Total Fitness, and earning a spot on *Men's Journal*'s "Top 100 Fitness Trainers in America" list. He began his lifelong dedication to health and fitness in Europe as a distinguished martial artist.

After coming to the United States, Samir began his career with the largest fitness organization at the time—Bally Total Fitness, initially as a fitness trainer and finally as a senior director responsible for the largest Bally's facility in America and four other clubs. He left the organization in 2009 to start ReSYNC Enterprises and *Health Fitness Revolution* online magazine, which has now become one of the fastest-growing health and fitness websites in America.

Samir has served as the fitness adviser for H-E-B, the largest grocery chain in Texas, and he regularly writes a column for the prestigious German news magazine *Focus*. He regularly speaks at corporate and nonprofit events and is frequently featured, quoted, or referenced in media across the world.

In addition, he developed the fitness program for Joel Osteen's Lakewood Church, which has the largest congregation in the United States, and has been a fitness consultant to many other religious and corporate groups as well.

Samir lives in Houston, Texas, with his wife, Dijana, and son, Ares Max.

Notes

Chapter 1: The Mission: To ReSYNC Your Body, Brain, and Spirit for a Longer, Healthier Life

1. MK McGovern, "The Effects of Exercise on the Brain," Serendip Studio, Spring 2005, http://serendip.brynmawr.edu/bb/neuro/neuro05/web2/mmcgovern.html.
2. J. C. Coulson, J. McKenna, and M. Field, "Exercising at Work and Self-Reported Work Performance," *International Journal of Workplace Health Management* 1, no. 3 (2008): 176–97, doi:10.1108/17538350810926534.
3. Harold G. Koenig, "Religion, Spirituality, and Health: The Research and Clinical Implications," *International Scholarly Research Notices: Psychiatry*, December 16, 2012, doi:10.5402/2012/278730.
4. Ibid.
5. Ibid.
6. Shanshan Li, "Association of Religious Service Attendance with Mortality Among Women," *JAMA Internal Medicine* 176, no. 6 (2016): 777–85, doi:10.1001/jamainternmed.2016.1615.
7. Lisa Miller et al., "Neuroanatomical Correlates of Religiosity and Spirituality: A Study in Adults at High and Low Familial Risk for Depression," *JAMA Psychiatry* 71, no. 2 (2014): 128–35, doi:10.1001/jamapsychiatry.2013.3067.

Chapter 2: ReSYNC Your Body: Twenty-Eight Days to Strong

1. Harvard Medical School, "Is It Okay to Be Fat If You're Fit?" Harvard Health Publications, May 2005, http://www.health.harvard.edu/staying-healthy /is-it-okay-to-be-fat-if-youre-fit.

2. Harvard Medical School, "Higher Cardio Fitness May Improve Multitasking Skills," Harvard Health Publications, February 2016, http://www.health.harvard. edu/exercise-and-fitness/higher-cardio-fitness-may-improve-multitasking-skills.

3. Benjamin L. Willis et al., "Midlife Fitness and the Development of Chronic Conditions in Later Life," *JAMA Internal Medicine* 172, no. 17 (2012): 1333–40, doi:10.1001/archinternmed.2012.3400.

Chapter 3: ReSYNC Your Diet: Twenty-Eight Days to Lean and Healthy

1. Jason Allen Mayberry, "Scurvy and Vitamin C," LEDA at Harvard Law School, Winter 2004, https://dash.harvard.edu/bitstream/handle/1/8852139/Mayberry .html?sequence=2.

2. Ashley Pierson, "Does Drinking Water Help Curb Hunger?" SFGate, http://healthyeating.sfgate.com/drinking-water-curb-hunger-4001.html.

3. Michael Boschmann et al., "Water-Induced Thermogenesis," *Journal of Clinical Endocrinology and Metabolism* 88, no. 12 (2016): 6015–19, doi:10.1210 /jc.2003–030780.

4. Gina Shaw, "Water and Your Diet: Staying Slim and Regular with H2O," WebMD, http://www.webmd.com/diet/water-for-weight-loss-diet?page=2.

5. Kathleen M. Zelman, "6 Reasons to Drink Water," WebMD, http://www.webmd .com/diet/6-reasons-to-drink-water?page=2.

6. Matthew S. Ganio et al., "Mild Dehydration Impairs Cognitive Performance and Mood of Men," *British Journal of Nutrition* 106 (2011): 1535–43, doi:10.1017 /S0007114511002005.

7. Lawrence E. Armstrong et al., "Mild Dehydration Affects Mood in Healthy Young Women," *Journal of Nutrition*, December 21, 2011, doi:10.3945/jn.111.142000.

8. Janelle Commins, "USDA Recommended Daily Water Intake," LiveStrong.com, http://www.livestrong.com/article/355482-usda-recommended-daily-water-intake/.

9. Technical University of Denmark (DTU), "Food's Transit Time Through Body Is a Key Factor in Digestive Health," *ScienceDaily*, June 27, 2016, https://www .sciencedaily.com/releases/2016/06/160627125525.htm.

10. *Harvard Health Letter*, "Mindful Eating," Harvard Health Publications, February 2011, http://www.health.harvard.edu/staying-healthy/mindful-eating.

11. Tamara Duker Freuman, "Digestion vs. Metabolism: The Misunderstood Relationship Between Digestion and Metabolism," *U.S. News and World Report*, February 5, 2013, http://health.usnews.com/health-news/blogs/eat-run/2013/02/05/digestion-vs-metabolism.

12. Kris Gunnars, "Eggs and Cholesterol—How Many Eggs Can You Safely Eat?" Authority Nutrition, https://authoritynutrition.com/how-many-eggs-should-you-eat/.

13. H. J. Leidy, "Increased Dietary Protein Consumed at Breakfast Leads to an Initial and Sustained Feeling of Fullness During Energy Restriction Compared to Other Meal Time," *British Journal of Nutrition* 101, no. 6 (2009): 798–803, https://www.ncbi.nlm.nih.gov/pubmed/19283886.

14. M. Micallef et al., "Plasma n-3 Polyunsaturated Fatty Acids Are Negatively Associated with Obesity," *British Journal of Nutrition* 102, no. 9 (2009): 137–74, doi:10.1017/S0007114509382173.

15. Olivia I. Okereke et al., "Dietary Fat Types and 4-Year Cognitive Change in Community-Dwelling Older Women," *Annals of Neurology* 72, no. 1 (May 17, 2012): 124–34, doi:10.1002/ana.23593.

16. Tufts University, "Low-Carb Diets Can Affect Dieters' Cognition Skills," *ScienceDaily*, December 15, 2008, https://www.sciencedaily.com/releases/2008/12/081211112014.htm.

17. Jeffrey Norris, "Sugar Is a Poison, Says UCSF Obesity Expert," *UCSF News*, June 25, 2009, https://www.ucsf.edu/news/2009/06/8187/obesity-and-metabolic-syndrome-driven-fructose-sugar-diet.

18. Helpguide.org, "Vitamins and Minerals: Are You Getting What You Need?" https://www.helpguide.org/harvard/vitamins-and-minerals.htm.

19. Patrick J. Skerrett, "Vitamin B12 Deficiency Can Be Sneaky, Harmful," Harvard Health Publications, October 18, 2016, http://www.health.harvard.edu/blog/vitamin-b12-deficiency-can-be-sneaky-harmful-201301105780.

Chapter 4: ReSYNC Your Brain: Twenty-Eight Days to Smart

1. Robert H. Wilkins, "Neurosurgical Classic-XVII Edwin Smith Surgical Papyrus," Cyber Museum of Neurosurgery, http://www.neurosurgery.org/cybermuseum/pre20th/epapyrus.html.

2. *Stanford Encyclopedia of Philosophy*, s.v. "Alcmaeon," http://plato.stanford.edu /entries/alcmaeon/.

3. Kevin McGrew, quoted in Lauren Cox, "Five Experts Answer: Can Your IQ Change?" Live Science, February 9, 2012, http://www.livescience.com/36143-iq -change-time.html.

4. "Sixty-Nine Interesting Facts About the Human Brain," Random Facts, http://facts .randomhistory.com/human-brain-facts.html.

5. "Top Fifteen Brain Facts," Sommer + Sommer, http://www.sommer-sommer.com /brainfacts/the-top-15-brain-facts/.

6. "The Memory Can Contain Up to 1 Quadrillion Bits of Information," Green Area, http://greenarea.me/en/67385/the-memory-can-contain-up-to-1-quadrillion -bits-of-information/.

7. Christof Koch, "Does Size Matter—for Brains?" *Scientific American*, January 1, 2016, https://www.scientificamerican.com/article/does-size-matter-for-brains/.

8. Jim Holt, "Time Bandits," *New Yorker*, February 28, 2005, http://www.newyorker. com/magazine/2005/02/28/time-bandits-2.

9. Ariana Huffington, "Hemingway, Thoreau, Jefferson and the Virtues of a Good Long Walk," *Huffington Post*, August 29, 2013, www.huffingtonpost.com/arianna -huffington/hemingway-thoreau-jeffers_b_3837002.html/.

10. Marily Oppezzo and Daniel L. Schwartz, "Give Your Ideas Some Legs: The Positive Effect of Walking on Creative Thinking," *Journal of Experimental Psychology: Learning, Memory, and Cognition* 40, no. 4 (2014): 1142–52, http://www.apa.org /pubs/journals/releases/xlm-a0036577.pdf.

11. Ibid.

12. Sherry L. Willis et al., "Long-Term Effects of Cognitive Training on Everyday Functional Outcomes in Older Adults," *JAMA* 296, no. 23 (2006): 2805–14, doi:10.1001/jama.296.23.2805.

13. "Mental Exercise Helps Maintain Some Seniors' Thinking Skills," news release, National Institutes of Health, December 19, 2006, https://www.nih.gov/news-events /news-releases/mental-exercise-helps-maintain-some-seniors-thinking-skills.

14. Joe Verghese et al., "Leisure Activities and the Risk of Dementia in the Elderly," *New England Journal of Medicine* 348 (2003): 2508–16, doi:10.1056/NEJMoa022252.

15. "Einstein's Brain," Phys.org, http://phys.org/news/2005-01-einsteins-brain.html.

16. National Research Council (US) Committee on Aging Frontiers in Social Psychology, Personality, and Adult Developmental Psychology, *When I'm 64*, eds. L. L. Carstensen and C. R. Hartel (Washington, DC: National Academies Press, 2006), https://www.ncbi.nlm.nih.gov/books/NBK83766/.

17. Holt, "Time Bandits."

18. Kirk I. Erickson et al., "Exercise Training Increases Size of Hippocampus and Improves Memory," *Proceedings of the National Academy of Sciences* 108, no. 7 (2011): 3017–22, doi:10.1073/pnas.1015950108.

19. Heidi Goodman, "Regular Exercise Changes the Brain to Improve Memory, Thinking Skill," *Harvard Health Letter*, April 9, 2014, http://www.health.harvard.edu/blog /regular-exercise-changes-brain-improve-memory-thinking-skills-201404097110.

20. Stanley J. Colcombe et al., "Aerobic Exercise Training Increases Brain Volume in Aging Humans," *Journal of Gerontology* 61, no. 11 (2006): 1166–70, http://www .ncbi.nlm.nih.gov/pubmed/17167157.

21. Joshua Z. Willey et al., "Leisure-Time Physical Activity Associates with Cognitive Decline: The Northern Manhattan Study," *Neurology* 86, no. 20 (2016): 1897–1903, doi:10.1212/WNL.0000000000002582.

22. Timothy J. Schoenfield et al., "Physical Exercise Prevents Stress-Induced Activation of Granule Neurons and Enhances Local Inhibitory Mechanisms in the Dentate Gyrus," *Journal of Neuroscience* 33, no. 18 (2013): 7770–77, http://www.jneurosci .org/content/33/18/7770.

23. Helen S. Driver and Sheila R. Taylor, "Exercise and Sleep," *Sleep Medicine Reviews* 4, no. 4 (2000): 387–402, doi:10.1053/smrv.2000.0110.

24. Stephen M. Pribut, "A Healthy Mind in a Healthy Body: Mens Sana in Corpore Sano," *Dr. Pribut's Blog*, January 19, 2013, http://www.drpribut.com/wordpress /2013/01/a-healthy-mind-in-a-healthy-body-mens-sana-in-corpore-sano/.

25. Holt, "Time Bandits."

26. Martha Clare Morris, et al., "Dietary Fats and the Risk of Incident Alzheimer Disease," *JAMA Neurology* 60, no. 2 (2003): 194–200, doi:10.1001/archneur.60.2.194.

27. Stephen Ceci, "IQ to the Test," *Psychology Today*, July 1, 2001, https://www .psychologytoday.com/articles/200107/iq-the-test.

28. Yian Gu et al., "Mediterranean Diet and Brain Structure in a Multiethnic Elderly Cohort," *Neurology* 85, no. 20 (2015): 1744–51, http://dx.doi.org/10.1212 /WNL.0000000000002121.

29. Stephanie Watson, "Caffeine and a Healthy Diet May Boost Memory, Thinking Skills; Alcohol's Effect Uncertain," Harvard Health Publications, June 18, 2014, http://www.health.harvard.edu/blog/caffeine-healthy-diet-may-boost-memory -thinking-skills-alcohols-effect-uncertain-201406187219; emphasis added.

30. Elaine Schmidt, "This Is Your Brain on Sugar: UCLA Study Shows High-Fructose Diet Sabotages Learning, Memory," UCLA Newsroom, May 15, 2012, http://newsroom.ucla.edu/releases/this-is-your-brain-on-sugar-ucla-233992.

31. R. Krikoian et al., "Concord Grape Juice Supplementation and Neurocognitive Function in Human Aging," *Journal of Agricultural and Food Chemistry* 60, no. 23 (2012): 5736–42, doi:10.1021/jf300277g.

32. Shrikant Mishra and Kalpana Palanivelu, "The Effect of Curcumin (Turmeric) on Alzheimer's Disease: An Overview," *Annals of Indian Academy of Neurology* 11, no. 1 (2008): 13–19, doi:10.4103/0972–2327.40220.

33. John Bachman and Nick Tate, "Harvard Researchers: Chocolate Protects Against Alzheimer's," NewsMaxHealth, October 22, 2013, http://www.newsmax.com /Health/Health-News/chocolate-alzheimer-dementia-cocoa/2013/10/22/id/532369/.

34. University of California–Los Angeles, "Scientists Learn How Food Affects the Brain: Omega 3 Especially Important," *ScienceDaily*, July 11, 2008, https://www .sciencedaily.com/releases/2008/07/080709161922.htm.

35. Mark Hamer, Emmanuel Stamatakis, and Gita D. Mishra, "Television-and Screen-Based Activity and Mental Well-Being in Adults," *American Journal of Preventive Medicine* 38, no. 4 (2010): 375–80, doi:10.1016/j.amepre.2009.12.030.

36. The JAMA Network Journals, "How Much TV You Watch As a Young Adult May Affect Midlife Cognitive Function," *ScienceDaily*, December 2, 2015, https://www .sciencedaily.com/releases/2015/12/151202132515.htm.

37. Corrie Goldman, "This Is Your Brain on Jane Austen, and Stanford Researchers Are Taking Notes," Stanford News, September 7, 2012, http://news.stanford.edu /news/2012/september/austen-reading-fmri-090712.html.

38. Gregory Berns, quoted in Carol Clark, "A Novel Look at How Stories May Change the Brain," eScience Commons, December 17, 2013, http: //esciencecommons.blogspot.com/2013/12/a-novel-look-at-how-stories-may -change.html.

39. Daniel Pendick, "Mental Strain Helps Maintain a Healthy Brain," Harvard Health Publications, November 5, 2012, www.health.harvard.edu/blog /mental-strain-helps-maintain-a-healthy-brain-201211055495.

40. Ravi Mehta and Rui (Juliet) Zu, "Blue or Red? Exploring the Effect of Color on Cognitive Task Performances," *Science* 323, no. 5918 (2009): 1226–29, doi:10.1126 /science.1169144.

41. Gary W. Small et al., "Your Brain on Google: Patterns of Cerebral Activation During Internet Searching," *American Journal of Geriatric Psychiatry* 17, no. 2 (2009): 116–26, doi:10.1097/JGP.0b013e3181953a02.

42. Maria A. Aberg et al., "Cardiovascular Fitness Is Associated with Cognition in Young Adulthood," *Proceedings of the National Academy of Sciences* 106, no. 49 (December 8, 2009): 20906–11, doi:10.1073/pnas.0905307106.

43. "Seven Ways to Improve Your IQ," *Men's Health*, November 20, 2016, www.menshealth.co.uk/healthy/brain-training/seven-ways-to-improve-your-iq.

44. "Aromatherapy," Skills You Need, https://www.skillsyouneed.com/ps /aromatherapy.html.

45. Jenna Iacurci, "Listening to Classical Music Good for the Brain," Nature World News, March 13, 2015, http://www.natureworldnews.com/articles/13417/20150313 /listening-to-classical-music-good-for-the-brain.htm.

46. Richard Restak, "Laughter and the Brain," *American Scholar*, Summer 2013, https: //theamericanscholar.org/laughter-and-the-brain/#.

Chapter 5: ReSYNC Your Spirit: Twenty-Eight Days to Spiritual Balance

1. New Hope Ladies Bible Study, "Lesson Three: Walking," http://newhopeladies .weebly.com/lesson-three-walking.html.

2. Rachael Rettner, "The Truth About '10,000 Steps' a Day," LiveScience, March 7, 2014, https://www.livescience.com/43956-walking-10000-steps-healthy.html.

3. Tara Parker-Pope, "The Pedometer Test: Americans Take Fewer Steps," *Well* (blog), October 19, 2010, http://well.blogs.nytimes.com/2010/10/19/the-pedometer -test-americans-take-fewer-steps/?_r=0.

4. Jack Wellman, "What Did Jesus Eat? Popular Bible Foods in the Day of Jesus," *Christian Crier* (blog), January 16, 2014, http://www.patheos.com/blogs /christiancrier/2014/01/16/what-did-jesus-eat-popular-bible-foods-in-the-day -of-jesus/.

5. "Prophet Muhammad (PBUH): 9 Healthy Habits That Science Later Proved," The Daily Crisp, December 23, 2015, http://thedailycrisp.com /prophet-muhammad-pbuh-9-healthy-habits-that-science-later-proved/.

6. Barbara O'Brien, "The Life of the Buddha," About Religion, April 30, 2016, http://buddhism.about.com/od/lifeofthebuddha/a/buddhalife.htm.

7. Christopher Peterson, "When Did the Buddha Become Fat?" *Psychology Today*, July 17, 2012, https://www.psychologytoday.com/blog/the-good-life/201207 /when-did-the-buddha-become-fat.

8. "Who Is St. Nicholas?" St. Nicholas Center, http://www.stnicholascenter.org/pages /who-is-st-nicholas/.

9. "St. Nicholas, Santa Claus and Father Christmas," WhyChristmas.com, www.whychristmas.com/customs/fatherchristmas.shtml.

10. Krista C. Cline and Kenneth F. Ferraro, "Does Religion Increase the Prevalence

and Incidence of Obesity in Adulthood?" *Journal for the Scientific Study of Religion* 45, no. 2 (2006): 269–81, doi:10.1111/j.1468–5906.2006.00305.x.

11. B. Wipfli et al., "An Examination of Serotonin and Psychological Variables in the Relationship Between Exercise and Mental Health," *Scandinavian Journal of Medicine and Science in Sports* 21, no. 3 (2009): 474–81, doi:10.1111/j.1600–0838.2009.01049.x/full.

12. Piper Li, "What Kind of Exercise Reduces Cortisol Levels?" Livestrong.com, January 12, 2014, http://www.livestrong.com/article/533372-what-kind-of -exercise-reduces-cortisol-levels/.

13. Elaine Magee, "How Food Affects Your Moods," WebMD, http://www.webmd.com /food-recipes/how-food-affects-your-moods.

14. "Spirituality," University of Maryland Medical Center, http://umm.edu/health /medical/altmed/treatment/spirituality.

15. Robert Wood Johnson Foundation, "Sense of Community," *Culture of Health*, accessed June 17, 2017, http://www.cultureofhealth.org/en/taking-action/making -health-a-shared-value/sense-of-community.html.

16. Chaeyoon Lim and Robert D. Putnam, "Religion, Social Networks, and Life Satisfaction," *American Sociological Review* 75, no. 6 (2010): 914–33, doi:10.1177/0003122410386686.

17. Laura D. Kubzansky and Rebecca C. Thurston, "Emotional Vitality and Incident Coronary Heart Disease," *Archives of General Psychiatry* 64, no. 12 (2007): 1393– 1401, http://jamanetwork.com/journals/jamapsychiatry/fullarticle/482515.

18. "Bible Verses About Meditation," King James Version Online, https://www .kingjamesbibleonline.org/Bible-Verses-About-Meditation.

19. "What Is Meditation?," The World Community for Christian Meditation, http://wccm.org/content/what-meditation.

20. Bruce Demarest, *Satisfy Your Soul: Restoring the Heart of Christian Spirituality* (Colorado Springs: NavPress, 1999), 133.

21. Perla Kaliman et al., "Rapid Changes in Histone Deacetylases and Inflammatory Gene Expression in Expert Meditators," *Psychoneuroendocrinology* 40 (2014): 96–107, doi:10.1016/j.psyneuen.2013.11.004.

22. Jill Sakai, "Study Reveals Gene Expression Changes with Meditation," University of Wisconsin–Madison News, December 4, 2013, http://news.wisc.edu /study-reveals-gene-expression-changes-with-meditation/.

23. Eileen Luders et al., "The Unique Brain Anatomy of Meditation Practitioners: Alterations in Cortical Gyrification," *Frontiers in Human Neuroscience*, February 29, 2012, doi:10.3389/fnhum.2012.00034.

24. Elizabeth W. Dunn and Michael Norton, "Hello Stranger," *New York Times Sunday Review*, April 25, 2014, https://www.nytimes.com/2014/04/26/opinion/sunday/hello-stranger.html.

25. Katherine Zeratsky, "Get into the Habit of Trying New Things," Mayo Clinic, June 26, 2014, http://www.mayoclinic.org/healthy-lifestyle/nutrition-and-healthy-eating/expert-blog/get-into-the-habit-of-trying-new-things/bgp-20095803.

26. Laura J. Solomon and Esther D. Rothblum, "Academic Procrastination: Frequency and Cognitive-Behavioral Correlates," *Journal of Counseling Psychology* 31, no. 4 (1984): 503–9, doi:10.1037/0022–0167.31.4.503.

27. Gregory N. Bratman et al., "Nature Experience Reduces Rumination and Subgenual Prefrontal Cortex Activation," *Proceedings of the National Academy of Sciences* 112, no. 28 (2015): 8567–72, http://www.pnas.org/content/112/28/8567.abstract.

28. Melinda Wenner, "Smile! It Could Make You Happier," *Scientific American*, September 1, 2009, www.scientificamerican.com/article/smile-it-could-make-you-happier/.

29. Lisa Fields, "6 Ways Pets Can Improve Your Health," WebMD, http://www.webmd.com/hypertension-high-blood-pressure/features/6-ways-pets-improve-your-health.

30. "The Many Health Benefits of Dancing," Berkeley Wellness, November 20, 2014, www.berkeleywellness.com/fitness/active-lifestyle/article/many-health-benefits-dancing.

31. Susan Scutti, "Change Your Posture to Improve Your Mood, Memory, and 5 Other Aspects of Your Life," Medical Daily, June 24, 2014, http://www.medicaldaily.com/change-your-posture-improve-your-mood-memory-and-5-other-aspects-your-life-289724.

32. Ean Weichsel, "The Value of Celebration (or Why Rewarding Yourself Is So Important)," *Ean Weichselbaum* (blog), April 24, 2016, https://eanweichsel.wordpress.com/2016/04/24/the-value-of-celebration-or-why-rewarding-yourself-is-so-important/.

33. Sara Klein, "6 Ways Singing Is Surprisingly Beneficial to Your Health," *Prevention*, May 18, 2016, www.prevention.com/health/6-health-benefits-of-singing.

34. Dawn Gluskin, "7 Ways to Lift Your Spirits on a Bad Day," *HuffPost the Blog*, updated January 25, 2014, http://www.huffingtonpost.com/dawn-gluskin/bad-day_b_4293637.html.

35. "The Power of Love," *NIH News in Health*, February 2007, https://newsinhealth.nih.gov/2007/february/docs/01features_01.htm.

36. "Stress Relief from Laughter? It's No Joke," Mayo Clinic Healthy Lifestyle, www.mayoclinic.org/healthy-lifestyle/stress-management/in-depth/stress-relief/art-20044456.

37. Susan Krauss Whitbourne, "How Reading Can Change You in a Major Way," *Psychology Today*, January 6, 2015, https://www.psychologytoday.com/blog /fulfillment-any-age/201501/how-reading-can-change-you-in-major-way.

38. Manish Jha, "Art and Spirituality—Spreading Positive Energy," Manish Jha, http://manishjha.net/2015/02/25/art-and-spirituality-innovation/.

39. Ali Geary, "7 Ways to Improve Your Spiritual Wellness," Illinois State University News, February 26, 2014, https://news.illinoisstate.edu/2014/02/7-ways-improve -spiritual-wellness/ (site discontinued).

40. Jessica Cassity, "The 7 Most Powerful Ways to Boost Your Happiness Right Now," Happify Daily, https://www.happify.com/hd/most-powerful-ways-to-boost-happiness/.

41. Stephanie Watson, "Volunteering May Be Good for Body and Mind," Harvard Health Publications, June 26, 2013, http://www.health.harvard.edu/blog /volunteering-may-be-good-for-body-and-mind-201306266428.

Chapter 7: The Power of ReSYNCing for Life

1. Craig R. Whitney, "Jeanne Calment, World's Elder, Dies at 122," *New York Times*, August 5, 1997, http://www.nytimes.com/1997/08/05/world/jeanne-calment-world -s-elder-dies-at-122.html.

2. "Life Expectancy Increased by 5 Years Since 2000, but Health Inequalities Persist," news release, World Health Organization, May 19, 2016, http://www.who.int /mediacentre/news/releases/2016/health-inequalities-persist/en/.

3. Gregg Easterbrook, "What Happens When We All Live to 100?" *Atlantic*, October 2014, https://www.theatlantic.com/magazine/archive/2014/10/what-happens -when-we-all-live-to-100/379338/.

4. A. Ruiz-Torres and W. Beier, "On Maximum Human Life Span: Interdisciplinary Approach About Its Limits," *Advances in Gerontology* 16 (2005): 14–20. https://www.ncbi.nlm.nih.gov/pubmed/16075672.

5. H. Arem et al., "Leisure Time Physical Activity and Mortality: A Detailed Pooled Analysis of the Dose-Response Relationship," *JAMA Internal Medicine* 175, no. 6 (2015): 959–67, doi:10.1001/jamainternmed.2015.0533.

6. "Why Is Sleep Important?" National Institutes of Health, February 22, 2012, https://www.nhlbi.nih.gov/health/health-topics/topics/sdd/why.

7. Hans K Meier-Ewert et al., "Effect of Sleep Loss on C-Reactive Protein, an Inflammatory Marker of Cardiovascular Risk," *Journal of the American College of Cardiology* 43, no. 4 (2004): 678–83, doi:10.1016/j.jacc.2003.07.050.

8. Michael J. Breus, "Sleep Habits: More Important Than You Think," Web MD, http://www.webmd.com/sleep-disorders/features/important-sleep-habits.

9. Harvard School of Public Health, "Sleep Deprivation and Obesity," Nutrition Source, https://www.hsph.harvard.edu/nutritionsource/sleep/.

10. Eve Van Cauter et al., "The Impact of Sleep Deprivation on Hormones and Metabolism," Medscape, http://www.medscape.org/viewarticle/502825.

11. Joseph Mercola, "Want a Good Night's Sleep? Then Never Do These Things Before Bed," Mercola, October 2, 2010, http://articles.mercola.com/sites/articles /archive/2010/10/02/secrets-to-a-good-night-sleep.aspx.

12. University of North Carolina at Chapel Hill, "Social Networks As Important As Exercise, Diet Across the Span of Our Lives: Researchers Show How Social Relationships Reduce Health Risk in Each Stage of Life," *ScienceDaily*, January 4, 2016, https://www.sciencedaily.com/releases/2016/01/160104163210.htm.

13. Julianne Holt-Lunstad et al., "Social Relationships and Mortality Risk: A Meta-Analytic Review," *PLOS Medicine* 7, no. 7 (2010): e1000316, http://journals.plos.org /plosmedicine/article?id=10.1371/journal.pmed.1000316.

14. "Spirituality May Help People Live Longer," WebMD, http://www.webmd.com /balance/features/spirituality-may-help-people-live-longer.

15. University of Colorado at Boulder, "Research Shows Religion Plays a Major Role in Health, Longevity," ScienceDaily, May 17, 1999, https://www.sciencedaily.com /releases/1999/05/990517064323.htm.